SHAMANIC PLANT MEDICINE
Salvia Divinorum: The Sage of the Seers

SHAMANIC PLANT MEDICINE

Salvia Divinorum: The Sage of the Seers

Ross Heaven

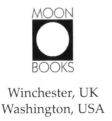

Winchester, UK
Washington, USA

First published by Moon Books, 2014
Moon Books is an imprint of John Hunt Publishing Ltd., Laurel House, Station Approach,
Alresford, Hants, SO24 9JH, UK
office1@jhpbooks.net
www.johnhuntpublishing.com
www.moon-books.net

For distributor details and how to order please visit the 'Ordering' section on our website.

Text copyright: Ross Heaven 2013

ISBN: 978 1 78279 252 9

A CIP catalogue record for this book is available from the British Library.

Design: Stuart Davies

Printed and bound by CPI Group (UK) Ltd, Croydon, CR0 4YY

We operate a distinctive and ethical publishing philosophy in all
areas of our business, from our global network of authors to
production and worldwide distribution.

CONTENTS

For Bodge (who else), the unsung and unseen Salvia hero, for the kids and for Indie.

About the Author

Ross Heaven is the author of several books on shamanism, plant teachers and healing and runs workshops on these themes in Europe and Peru, including Shamanic Practitioner training programmes; Shamanic Healing and Soul Retrieval courses; plant medicine retreats with San Pedro, Salvia and ayahuasca, and journeys to Peru to work with indigenous shamans. He is also a shamanic healer and therapist and offers counselling, soul retrieval and healing in the UK.

He has a website at www.thefourgates.org where you can read more about his work as well as forthcoming books and other items of interest. He also provides a monthly newsletter by e-mail, which you can receive free of charge by emailing ross@thefourgates.org.

His other books on plant teachers and medicines include *Cactus of Mystery, The Hummingbird's Journey to God* and *Drinking the Four Winds* (about San Pedro), *Plant Spirit Shamanism* (about ayahuasca and Amazonian plant healing) and *The Sin Eater's Last Confessions* (about Celtic methods of soul healing with herbs and plants). Others in the Shamanic Plant Medicine series include *Ayahuasca, San Pedro* and *Sacred Mushrooms*. His full book list can be viewed at Amazon Books.

Shamanic Plant Medicine
The first practical guide to working with teacher plants

Shamanic Plant Medicine is a series of books written to provide you with a succinct and practical introduction to a specific teacher or power plant, its history, shamanic uses, healing applications and benefits, as well as the things to be aware of when working with these plants, including ceremonial procedures and safety precautions. These plants are also known in the Western world as entheogens: substances which 'reveal the God within', and in shamanic cultures as allies: helpful spirits which confer power and pass on insights and information.

The first in this series are *Ayahuasca: The Vine of Souls, San Pedro: The Gateway to Wisdom, Salvia Divinorum: The Sage of the Seers* and *Sacred Mushrooms: Messengers of the Stars.* It is a series which reveals the truth about these plants and provides an insight into their uses as well as the cautions to take with them, so you are properly informed of your choices not reliant on sensationalism and disinformation.

The shamanic use of plants and herbs is one of the world's oldest healing methods and, despite propaganda to the contrary, it is usually the safest and most effective form of medicine too.

In 2005, for example, the British Medical Journal warned that 'in England alone reactions to drugs that led to hospitalisation followed by death are estimated at 5,700 a year and could actually be closer to 10,000.' By comparison, between 2000 and August 2004 there were just 451 reports of adverse reactions to herbal preparations and only 152 were considered serious. No fatalities. That statistic equates to just 38 problem cases a year resulting from plant medicines compared to perhaps 10,000 deaths a year as a result of accepted mainstream medicine. Reviewing these figures the London Independent newspaper concluded that, 'Herbs may not be completely safe as critics like to point out – but they are a lot safer than drugs.'

The situation in America is very similar. Here, orthodox medical treatment itself is now the leading cause of death, ahead of heart disease and cancer, and 'Infections, surgical mistakes and other medical harm contributes to the deaths of 180,000 hospital patients a year [and] another 1.4 million are seriously hurt by their hospital care.' (Consumer Reports online: www.consumer-reports.org). Other studies reveal that adverse drug reactions are under-reported by up to 94 percent since the US government does not adequately track them. Death as a result of plant healings meanwhile remain next to zero.

It is worth asking why these figures so often go unreported, and why the medical profession continues to treat people as it does, even with full awareness of the risks and comparisons. Another good question would be why plants and herbs more than drugs and orthodox medicine are the focus of governments for stricter regulation (see for example the current *codex alimentarius* proposals) despite their effectiveness and comparative freedom from risk. Who benefits?

More remarkable even than their ability to heal the body is the ability of some plants to expand the mind, raise consciousness, release stuck or damaging emotions and connect us more deeply to spirit. These are the teacher plants. By showing us our true power and potential they enable us to see through illusions and explore the real nature of the dreaming universe so we discover our purpose on Earth.

Plant teachers are used by shamans the world over in a sacred ritual context to divine the future, enter spirit realms, learn the deepest truths of themselves and the universe (although many shamans see little distinction between the two since, as they say, 'the world is as you dream it'; that is, each of us *is* the universe).

They also enable them – and us – to perform true healings which go beyond the abilities of modern medicine and its reliance on intrusive treatments and often damaging drugs.

Salvia Divinorum: The Sage of the Seers

There was much of the beautiful, much of the wanton, much of the bizarre, something of the terrible, and not a little of that which might have excited disgust.
Edgar Allan Poe, *The Masque of the Red Death*

1

Salvia and Salvinorin A
'It is Total Madness... Tearing Apart the Fabric of Reality'

She is either not alive or not terrestrial...
We knew then that she had come from another dimension
Bruce Rimmell, writing about the nature and origins of
Salvia

Salvia divinorum is the botanical name of a visionary plant used in shamanic rituals for healing and divination by the medicine men and *curanderos* (healers) of Oaxaca, Mexico, who are referred to in this region as *cho-ta-ci-ne*: 'one who knows'. In contemporary circles an extract of the plant, salvinorin A – widely regarded as the world's most powerful natural hallucinogen, up to 200 times stronger than LSD – is also gaining respect among shamans and seekers as an express route to self-discovery and the expansion of consciousness.

The genus name, Salvia, comes from the Latin *salvare*, to heal or to save, while its complete botanical name, also from the Latin, is generally understood as 'the sage of the seers'. The Mazatec shamans of Mexico, however, know it by less formal names, most of which are associated with the Virgin Mary who is seen as the embodiment of its spirit. Among them are ska Maria pastora (Mary the shepherdess), hojas de Maria (leaves of Mary), hojas de la pastora (leaves of the shepherdess), hierba Maria (Mary's herb), and, according to the psychedelic explorer Terence McKenna, at least, as ojos de la pastora (the eyes of the shepherdess).

In traditional shamanic usage the fresh leaves are rolled and chewed as a quid or made into a tea and drunk. Taken in this way the effects are usually mild, producing a dreamy, trance-like, somewhat euphoric state and the ability to tune in empathically to people around you or to your environment. It is not always this gentle, however, as the anthropologist Bret Blosser writes, about an experience he had in Mexico in the 1980s where the effects were somewhat stronger: 'I never noticed the transition. I was not aware that I had eaten an entheogenic plant, was in Mexico, was with friends, or had ever had a body. I was engulfed in a complex, fluctuating environment...

'Toward the end I recall an intricate, neon-pastel, slick-lit, all encompassing, non-Euclidian topography. This sense of a distinctive topography has characterized each of my Mazatec Salvia experiences. Of course, what I can describe begs the question of what I cannot describe: *being out of the three dimensions and linear time.*' (My italics).

It is the active ingredient, however – salvinorin A – which, when vaporised and inhaled or smoked in a pipe (the more frequent way of working with Salvia these days), delivers the more potent experience. This is usually complex and deep (while also paradoxically simple and direct in the lessons it gives us), quickly and intensely shredding the veil which human beings have drawn over the nature of 'true reality' (whatever that may actually mean) and plunging the smoker into a strange and alien landscape where the answers he finds, while so incredible and shocking that he may almost wish they had remained hidden, have the ring of authentic and absolute truth.

Among these lessons are these:

- That the world is not real
- That *we* are not real (and nor is most of what we *think* we know about ourselves)
- That we are the creators of the world, filled with power and potential, but that we are also created and at the whim of alien gods

- That there is no cause and effect (A does not lead to B), but that the process of life is a karmic circle where we get back in equal measure exactly what we have put out
- That time and space do not exist
- That there are other dimensions around us which we are also a part of and which influence our lives in unseen ways and, most strangely of all
- That human beings may actually be a construct, a game that is being played by an intelligence greater than ours which we have no way of knowing

These discoveries – as you will see later in this book – may cause those who some Salvia to question not only their sanity but the nature of our entire existence and the universe which we have – until now – believed that we occupied, because the truth that Salvia gives us – in the words of Theodore Roszak, author of the book *Flicker* – is that, 'We live as film, on a film, the skin of a bubble. What is real lives behind, waiting to push through, swallow us up, reclaim us. It may not be nice.'

While absolutely profound and real, that is, these insights and conclusions are not always easy or pleasant for those who emerge with Salvia's answers. But if you really want to know the truth of the world you live in – as all shamans and seekers must – there is no faster route to this knowledge, or a more direct teacher.

The Plant and its History

Despite its name, *sage* of the seers, Salvia is actually an herb in the mint family. It can be cultivated and grown in many warm and humid places in the world, although it originates from a very specific location in the forests of the Sierra Mazateca, Mexico, at altitudes of between 750 and 1,500 metres. It can reach a metre in height and has large green leaves, hollow square stems, and white flowers with purple calyces.

Its use by Mazatec shamans is not well documented and, in contrast to the ritual use of psilocybin ('magic') mushrooms in this region, and peyote in other parts of Mexico, both of which had been recorded from as early as the sixteenth century, information on Salvia is also much more recent, dating only from the 1930s. One of the first references comes from Jean Johnson, an American anthropologist who discovered in 1938 that Mazatec shamans used a tea made from Salvia leaves in a manner similar to the mushrooms, for divination when the latter were out of season.

In 1952 Roberto Weitlaner reported on the plant, writing that an infusion of 50 leaves was normally used by shamans in healing ceremonies which took place at midnight in a dark room where the patient drank the potion. After about fifteen minutes he would enter a trance and from his descriptions of his visions the healer was able to make a diagnosis of the cause of his illness and know how to cure it. The session ended by bathing the patient in some of the same infusion he had drunk.

Gordon Wasson was the first to describe the Salvia experience, after a ceremony in 1961 where he drank the juice of 34 pairs of leaves (68 in total). He noted that the effects came on faster than those of mushrooms although they lasted a much shorter time, and reported seeing colours and three-dimensional designs. The first Salvia specimens were also collected by Wasson, along with Weitlaner and Albert Hofmann (the discoverer of LSD). They drank the brew together in 1962 and Hofmann said his experience was intense and created a state of heightened 'mental sensitivity' although it did not result in 'hallucinations'. His wife, who accompanied him and also drank, reported seeing bright images.

Jose Diaz studied Salvia in the Mazatec highlands during the 1970s and 80s, drinking an infusion of the plant on six occasions and noting that its potency increased each time. He saw patterns which he described as 'complex and slowly changing' and felt lightness in his arms and legs and an 'odd sensation' in his joints, which lasted about ten minutes although more subtle effects continued for hours.

Wasson, Diaz and Richard Evans Schultes also studied the shamans of Mexico, all of them remarking on the difficulty of making contact with them and gathering information because of what Diaz called their 'jealous and secretive nature'. Despite this Diaz was able to find one shaman, *don* Alejandro,[1] from whom he was able to gather information during fieldwork in the summer of 1979 and spring of 1980.

Diaz learned that training to become a shaman is through an apprenticeship which lasts for two or more years and teaches the practicalities of healing. Teacher plants are taken at intervals of a week to a month with spiritual instruction coming through the visions these produce and the teachings of 'angelic beings'. The process begins with successively increasing doses of Salvia which are said to familiarise the shaman with the route to Heaven where healing may be found.

In common with all plant work, a strict diet is followed during this training,[2] with spicy foods such as chilli prohibited and abstinence from sex and alcohol, although Diaz remarks that some shamans allow the drinking of beer, and tequila may be consumed in a ritual context. The first Salvia diet lasts for sixteen days with subsequent diets for a minimum of four days. Breaking it can lead to madness.

The shaman is taught that Salvia can be used as a medicine as well as for visions. For example a tea made from five pairs of leaves will cure anaemia, headaches, rheumatism and stomach problems. There is also a magical disease that is cured by Salvia, which is known as *panzón de borrego* ('lamb belly') and takes the form of a swollen stomach which results from a curse made by a *brujo* (sorcerer) who has placed a stone inside the sufferer. Salvia removes it so the stomach returns to normal.

Aside from healing, Salvia is used for divination and for this purpose it is prepared as an infusion of 20 to 80 pairs of fresh leaves which may be taken by the curandero, the patient, or both depending on the situation. Salvia will then foretell the future and provide answers to detailed questions.

The observation that '20 to 80 pairs' of leaves are used comes from Diaz, but it is not very useful. There is a 60-pair (120-leaf) difference between these extremes, which is a pretty wide margin. To add to the confusion Christian Rätsch in *The Encyclopedia of Psychoactive Plants* writes that, 'The Mazatec take thirteen pairs of fresh leaves (twenty-six leaves in all) and roll them into a kind of cigar (quid) that they place in the mouth and suck on or chew ... At least six fresh leaves are needed to prepare one quid (threshold dosage), while more distinct effects will occur with eight to ten leaves...

'Dried leaves are best smoked by themselves. Here as little as half an average-sized leaf (two or three deep inhalations) can be sufficient to elicit profound psychoactive effects. Usually however one or two leaves are smoked ...

'Tinctures are prepared from fresh or dried leaves by using an ethanol-water mixture (60 per cent alcohol)... Dosages appear to vary considerably...'

According to this, Salvia can therefore be drunk as a tea, chewed, smoked, or held in the mouth as a tincture and not just in the way (or in the quantity) that Diaz describes. In modern usage the extract can also be smoked in a pipe or vaporised and inhaled. There seems to be little standardisation then, even among shamans in traditional ceremonial contexts, as to how – or how much – Salvia is taken. As the ethnopharmacologist Karl Mayer remarks, 'To date little that is certain is known about the Salvia ritual as corresponding ethnographic or historical evidence is lacking.'

To deal with this confusion at the outset for people who may want to try Salvia themselves, I have found that an infusion of 60 dried leaves (30 pairs) added to approximately half a pint of hot water works well (leave it to soak overnight and drink it first thing, when it is cold). If chewed as a quid, the same number of fresh or pre-soaked leaves are held between the teeth and gums for about fifteen minutes so that the active ingredient passes into the bloodstream. When smoked, four or five pairs (eight to ten) of dried leaves can be crumbled into a pipe and some people say that two or three pipes, one after the other, produce more dramatic, salvinorin-like effects. More usually, however, I use the leaves as a base for the extract itself.

Salvia Ceremonies

One thing the literature does agree on is that Salvia ceremonies almost always take place at night or in complete darkness and silence because, according to Rätsch, 'Both sounds and sources of light will greatly disturb the visionary experience.' In my experience too, darkness, silence, intention (i.e. a purpose to the ceremony – to gather information, answer a question, solve a problem or see the future) and, as much as is possible, a continued focus on that intention *do* aid the journey and help us to make sense of it afterwards.

In the ceremonies Diaz attended, the *curandero* (healer) made the infusion as night fell, with the leaves counted in pairs and put into piles before being crushed by hand into a bowl of water. The potion was then sieved into a glass and the spent leaves set aside to bathe the participant's head and revive him after the ceremony. The curandero then called upon the Holy Trinity, the Virgin Mary, Saint Peter and other saints to watch over partici-pants. The participants drank the brew as the shaman performed *limpias* (ritual cleansings) on them by reciting prayers and anointing them with a piece of copal dipped in tobacco juice.

During his first ceremony conducted in this way, Diaz drank an infusion made from 50 pairs of leaves and after about fifteen minutes began to see visions, like columns of smoke in the darkness; then as the images increased in intensity, a mountain of ice, lights of various colours, a dark sky with bright objects in it, and a native village. The session lasted about an hour.

In his second session he drank an infusion of 60 pairs of leaves and after fifteen minutes again felt the effects of Salvia: a sense of relaxation and colourful images of plants and flowers. A little later he reported that, 'I feel like I'm being twisted around inside of my body. Very strange sensations ... like I'm spinning.' He also recalled seeing 'a large boat or something like that.[3] And as if all the things inside were all very mechanical, like a machine that was very, very precise and very geometric... And again I began to see many flowers, but as if they were all mechanical, as if they were not ... real.' These sensations of being twisted or pulled and visions of things mechanical, of being inside a machine and of reality being not quite 'real' are characteristic of the Salvia experience as you will see.

Don Alejandro encouraged Diaz and his companions to talk about their visions throughout the ceremony and afterward in order to clarify them, although this seems less common among other curanderos where ritual use involves silence so that the plant itself can be heard (Mazatec shamans say that 'La Maria speaks with a quiet voice'). For many who have taken Salvia (especially in extract form) the immediate effects can be so extraordinary that they *do* wish to talk, if only to reconnect with the 'normal' world, but this is to risk prematurely deconstructing their journey or becoming so caught up in their descriptions that they do not hear the information that may still be being passed to them by the plant. In my experience the more useful insights and realisations tend to arise during the 30 minutes or so *after* the peak experience (or it may come in dreams following the ceremony that night) and continued silence is needed to hear them.

Salvinorin A, the Extract and its History

The 'active ingredient' of Salvia, Salvinorin A, was first isolated from the plant by Alfredo Ortega in 1982 although he did not investigate its psychoactive properties. Another group led by Leander Valdes III did, his results confirming that salvinorin A was the visionary component although it was only tested on lab animals (mice) not on humans.

Human testing came in 1993 with the work of Daniel Siebert who was the first to produce concentrated extracts and explore their effects by smoking them. His first encounter with the essence of Salvia was strange and dramatic and, as much as anything, describes the sort of experience that is common when smoking the extract: mind-blowing, world-shaking and, for some, terrifying, but also deeply illuminating.

Quite suddenly I found myself in a confused, fast-moving state of consciousness with absolutely no idea where my body or, for that matter, my universe had gone.

I have little memory of this initial period of the experience but I do know that a lot was happening and that it seemed quite literally like an eternity when in fact it must only have lasted a few minutes. I wanted desperately to get back to the 'real' world. I searched my memory trying to remember the living room I was sitting in just moments before. I tried to remember what my body felt like. Anything. Just something to reconnect me with the 'normal' world. But the more I looked for some little thread of 'normality' to get a hold of, the more it showed me something else.

At some point I realized that what I was trying to get back to did not exist. It was just an ephemeral dream. I suddenly realized that I had no actual memory of ever having lived in any other state of consciousness but the disembodied condition I was now in... I was totally convinced that this state of existence was all there ever was... Apparently, had I so willed it, I could return to any point in my life and *really be there* because it was actually happening *right now*...

13

A little later the physical world all started to work properly again... I grabbed a pen and tried to write down a few notes while the experience was still fresh. The first thing I wrote down in big letters was: IT IS TOTAL MADNESS, then: [it is] TEARING APART THE FABRIC OF REALITY... I had been shaken to the soul.

Dr Bryan Roth agrees with Siebert about the potency of the extract. In 2002 he discovered that salvinorin A, uniquely, stimulates a single receptor site in the brain, the kappa opioid. LSD by comparison stimulates about 50 receptors to produce its effects which, even then, are not as potent or immediate. 'Dr Roth said salvinorin A was the strongest hallucinogen gram for gram found in nature,' the New York Times reported.

Longer-term Salvia Effects

The Salvia (Salvinorin) 'trip' itself may only last a few minutes (my own longest journey was around 25-30 minutes and that was at one of the highest concentrations of the extract), followed by a recommended period of reintegration and reflection for 30 minutes or so, so about an hour in all. Even after it ends, however, there may in fact be other more subtle effects which are on-going if attention is paid to them, and which are generally regarded as beneficial. Researchers from the University of California and California Pacific Medical Center Research Institute conducted a survey of 500 Salvia users, for example, which showed effects that could last for days. They included:

- Increased insight (47 percent of subjects)
- Improved mood (44.8 percent)
- Calmness (42.2 percent) and, significantly – for me and my own participants in Salvia ceremonies, at least
- 'Weird thoughts' (36.4 percent) and
- 'Things seeming unreal' (32.4 percent)

It is a pity that the word 'weird' was not better defined in this research. The results of my own experiments, however, would translate it to mean something like 'more creative and unconventional thinking', 'a new ability to see outside the box' or 'a new capacity to cut through the illusions, untruths and unreality of mainstream ideas and beliefs'.

Beyond this, Salvia may have even longer-term therapeutic potential. Professor Bryan Roth believes, for example, that drugs derived from the plant could help to combat Alzheimer's disease, depression, schizophrenia, chronic pain, and AIDS. Thomas Prisinzano, assistant professor of medicinal and natural products chemistry at the University of Iowa, suggests that Salvia may also help treat addictions: 'You can give a rat free access to cocaine [then] give them free access to salvinorin A, and they stop taking cocaine,' he says. Clinical pharmacologist John Mendelsohn summarises the research so far, that, 'There are a lot of therapeutic targets [for Salvia] that have many people excited.' Among others are eating disorders, motion sickness, hypertension, arrhythmia, multiple sclerosis, leukaemia, Type 1 diabetes, Epstein-Barr virus, cytomegalovirus and heroin, cocaine, alcohol and amphetamine dependency.

Salvia and Salvinorin: Initial Teachings

We can already begin to see some of the teachings of Salvia, and get some idea of what may be so unnerving about the experience of it, especially for those who smoke the extract for the first time: it takes us wholly – mind, body and spirit – out of the 'normal' world and, when we return (*if*, perhaps, we return at all to the same world we left), forces us to question the very foundations of that world; for what, after all, is 'normal' or 'real'? For most of us it is what we have been told by others to accept unquestioningly as true, and yet there are mysteries in even our most basic assumptions about ourselves and the universe. Salvia brings us face-to-face with these mysteries and with the realisation that, not only are *we* not who we thought we were, but the world itself does not exist in the way we thought it did – if it exists at all.

More than any other plant I have worked with,[4] Salvia is a Zen master, revealing the paradoxes of life, the great uncertainty we move within, and the unknowable-ness of anything except at its most blunt and least interesting level; the lack of a fundamental and immutable 'truth', that is, to any 'reality' we think we may occupy.

In the normal world, for example, most of us, when asked our views of life, are likely to come down in favour of one or the other of society's majority worldviews: the side of *faith-without-evidence*, which asks us to accept that an unknown creator-God/Goddess/alien Prometheus is responsible for life on Earth, or the side of *evidence-without-faith*, which asks us to accept (also as an act of faith, paradoxically, since it has no real proof to offer either) that science has all the answers and that life – as 'miraculous' and unlikely as it may be – is the result of a happy accident, a random collision of amino acids and swamp gas, and Darwin took care of the rest. In other words, we are either of a scientific or a theological/philosophical persuasion. But that may only be because those are the only two options that our upbringing and education have given us. And what if they are both wrong? Perhaps the truth of life is even stranger and more unsettling: not just that there is no God or that science does not have the answers it claims to, but that life – *we*, in fact – does not even exist?

The problem for both camps – and for us, if we wish to look at our human condition and develop a more honest understanding about life and the universe – is that neither science nor religion can satisfactorily explain how something was created from nothing. Religion talks about God's will and the 'creative breath of life'; science talks about the 'big bang'. But neither offers us *proof* of its beliefs, simply because it can't. It is a difficulty which has led some scientists, like David Kaufmann of the University of

Florida, to remark that, 'Evolution lacks a scientifically acceptable explanation of the source of the precisely planned codes within cells, without which there can be no specific proteins and hence no life.' (In plain language, they haven't got a clue how life came to be.) It also led some philosophers, like professor Anthony Flew, to conclude that, 'A super-intelligence is the only good explanation for the origin of life.' By which he means a *non-human* intelligence (or, at least, not human as we know human beings today); a view, incidentally, that was shared by Francis Crick, the Nobel Prize winner for his discovery of DNA, and by many other scientists today.

And yet some of us are still willing to accept the limitations imposed on us by the belief systems of religion and science and even fight to the death to defend them when they have no substance at all. As the character Christof remarks in the film *The Truman Show*, 'We accept the reality with which we are presented.' In the absence of answers we have agreed to live by the pretences of others without even giving thought to the questions.

This is the type of unveiling that Salvia enjoys: the throwing of our cosy assumptions out of a metaphysical window. What is unnerving for some, then, is not the Salvia experience *per se* (in the sense of a 'bad trip' or being out of control, although the latter is certainly a part of most Salvia journeys) but the realisation that they are in fact not in control of their '*normal*' lives; that they are no-one and nothingness; that they have no answers. On top of that is often the understanding that, far from standing at the centre of creation at the top of the food chain, human beings are in fact unimportant – irrelevant even – to the universe (*if* such a thing even truly exists) and that life itself is meaningless.

Salvia takes us to a void, a quantum paradox: a nothing filled with everything where reality is anything we want it to be and nothing like we expected. In some ways then, the spirit of the plant is a scientist as well as a shaman, offering proof of time travel, alternative universes, other dimensions, karma and chaos, and in this it is not a million miles away from the seemingly crazy but disturbingly congruent findings of new physics whose current conclusions about human life is that we, as we understand ourselves, at least, do not exist. Instead, we are constructs, computer simulations, characters in a game. As Niels Bohr remarked: 'Anyone who is not shocked by quantum theory has not understood it.' The world of Salvia is much the same.

The idea that human life is a computer simulation comes from a 2003 paper in Philosophical Quarterly by Nick Bostrom, a philosophy professor at the University of Oxford. In it, he argues that the human race will probably become extinct before reaching a 'posthuman' stage but that any surviving civilisation is likely to run simulations of its history to understand where it came from – a not too incredible idea since we do something similar even today, for our amusement rather than education, in constructs like *The Sims* and *Second Life* where we become fantasy characters and play out our lives in a digital world. Bostrom concludes that, 'We are almost certainly living in a computer simulation.' All of us. Now.[5]

The idea sounds like a scene from *The matrix*...

Morpheus: The Matrix is everywhere, it is all around us. Even now in this very room. You can see it when you look out your window or when you turn on your television. You can feel it when you go to work or to church or when you pay your taxes. It is the world that has been pulled over your eyes to blind you from the truth.

Neo: What truth?

Morpheus: That you are... born inside a prison that you cannot smell, taste or touch. A prison for your mind.

Furthermore, as Morpheus goes on, 'No one can be told what the

Matrix is' – you cannot escape a lie by being told you are living it when you yourself are a part of that lie! 'You have to see it for yourself.' And this is what Salvia does. It's a bit like taking the red pill.

If Bostrom's idea was just a thought experiment it might be shocking enough if we allowed its ramifications to really sink in. But it is not. Quantum scientists have discovered evidence for it in the form of computer code written into the very fabric of the universe.

James Gates (professor of Physics, University of Maryland): Computer code. Strings of bits of ones and zeros.

Somewhat incredulous journalist: It not just *resembles* computer code? You're saying it *is* computer code?

Gates: It not only *is* computer code, it's a special kind of computer code… that's what we find buried very deeply inside [there].[6]

Salvia is the truth laid bare and a shortcut to the same quantum conclusions (see the participant accounts later in this book). That is what is most challenging about it for some, because its implications cannot be trivialised. It means, for example, that everything you hold most dear – the opinions you have, the campaigns you support, the issues that drive you, the principles you live by, the loves of your life – are all illusions and meaningless in themselves because they were never yours to begin with. You and they are simply plotlines and characters in someone else's drama.

The philosophical concerns underlying all of this – for example, freewill versus determinism: what we can change (if anything) about ourselves and our world, or how we can heal (if at all) – also raise practical 'real life' questions. Like: Who am I *really* if I have been pre-programmed to think and act as I do? Is change possible at an individual or global level? Who – or what

– is our 'creator', our God or our programmer? Is our survival and evolution possible, or is that up to somebody else? There are many other questions that arise too, about love and war and fate, but one of the most important, in the face of all of this, is 'How do I wish to live?' These are the questions that Salvia poses and the sort of research which is currently being conducted with this plant.

The Mystery of Salvia

If the universe were not mysterious enough, there are also mysteries to Salvia. Surprisingly, for example, the shamans of Mexico have no creation myths to explain its origin. This is unusual since with all other entheogens the personality of the teacher plant, its divine source and the reason for its gift to humankind are understood and described in myths which can often be traced back thousands of years.

The Huichol people of Mexico, for example, tell how the peyote cactus first arrived here with Tatewari (grandfather-fire), the oldest god, who is also known as Hikuri the peyote-god and is personified with peyote plants growing on his hands and feet. It was Tatewari who led the first peyote pilgrimage to Wirikuta, the ancestral region where the plant still grows. That was over 2,000 years ago but every year a select group of Huichols, usually ten to fifteen in number, walk the same route to gather peyote and follow Tatewari to 'find their life'.

With ayahuasca, the jungle medicine of the Amazon regions, legends tell that a shaman discovered the plant after a jealous deity cut the 'rope to the moon' which served as a connection between human beings and the divine. When this rope was severed what had been paradise on Earth became a world of sadness and anger and a shaman was instructed by his people to find a new rope so they could return to peace and happiness. In a vision the healer was told to walk into the jungle and 'turn two corners' and there he would find the plants he needed to rebuild the connection between worlds. At the beginning of time he did so, according to legend (or around 5,000 years ago, according to archaeologists who have discovered what are so far the earliest ritual artefacts used in ayahuasca ceremonies) and came upon the 'vine of souls' which we have been able to climb ever since to find paradise inside us.

The route to a better world was found by the shamans of the Andes, meanwhile, in San Pedro (*huachuma*), the mescaline cactus inside of which Saint Peter (San Pedro) hid the 'keys to Heaven'. It is said that the curanderos were led to it by following the flight of a hummingbird, its magical guardian spirit. Again, ritual artefacts and huachuma-inspired art show that this discovery was made over 3,500 years ago.

There are similar stories for other healing and teaching plants including mushrooms, cannabis and datura (the 'flying ointment' of witches) – but none at all for Salvia. As D M Turner writes in his book *Salvinorin: The Psychedelic Essence of Salvia Divinorum*, the Mazatecs even lack an indigenous name for Salvia, 'both the Christian theme of Mary, as well as sheep, having been introduced to the region during the Spanish conquest.' Furthermore, as he says, their method of consuming the plant (as a quid or a tea rather than a prepared extract) 'does not efficiently utilize its psychoactive content and [they] seem to be generally unaware of its tremendous potency'; a point echoed by the famous Mazatec shaman, Maria Sabina, who once remarked that, 'If I have a sick person during the season when mushrooms are not available I resort to the hojas de la Pastora... Of course, the Pastora doesn't have as much strength.' Something of an understatement when we are referring to the world's most potent natural hallucinogen.

Contemporary Western botanists have no answer for the origins of Salvia either and can't even say whether it is a naturally occurring species. The plant is partially sterile, which suggests a hybrid although no likely parent species have yet been found – but if that is the case it leads only to further questions; like who created it and why? Turner again: 'Salvia divinorum ... is not known to exist in the wild and the few patches that are known in the Sierra Mazateca appear to be the result of deliberate planting. A Mazatec shaman informed Wasson that the Indians believe the plant is foreign to their region and do not know from where it came. And if Salvia divinorum is a hybrid, there are no commonly held theories on what its prospective parents may be.'

A final puzzle is that no-one – scientist or shaman – seems to know quite how or why Salvia works. Although salvinorin A is the world's strongest natural hallucinogen, for example, it has no actions on the 5-HT_{2A} serotonin receptor, the principal molecular target for most psychedelics. Indeed, until Dr Bryan Roth's discovery in 2002 that it acts on the kappa opioid, it did not seem to have a target in the brain at all. Action on a single receptor site is still strange and unique, however, since other psychedelics require multiple targets.

These mysteries have led some people – again, scientists and shamans alike – to speculate that Salvia may not be indigenous to Earth at all. The artist Bruce Rimmell summarises the idea in his poem, *The Origin of Salvia Divinorum*:

> *we were scientists*
> *and we tested xca maria,*
> *took her leaves to our labs*
> *and examined and analysed*
> *til the sun was down...*
> *we found*
> *that she lacked dna,*
> *no genetic impulse at all...*
> *'she is either*
> *not alive*
> *or not terrestrial...'*

and we knew then
that she had come
from another dimension.
(i remember looking up to the sky
and wondering which star
she might have dropped from...)

Is Salvia a plant from another world, another universe or another dimension? The idea might be laughable except for the discoveries of quantum physics we looked at earlier: that there are other dimensions all around us and that we may ourselves be simulations created by entities from these other dimensions or by an alien intelligence or a future generation of 'posthumans' – which, on the face of it, sounds even crazier than the suggestion that a plant may have arrived here from another world. After all, one accepted theory of evolution is that life began on our planet when a comet crashed here from another, carrying microbes which, over millions of years, evolved into human beings. Why might a plant not have arrived in the same, or a similar, way?

And then there are the accounts of Salvia users and their journeys to destinations which seem anything but Earthly or human...

2

Salvia Origins and Teachings
'Strange News from Another Star'

We like to walk around sometimes and to see new places.
We like some of those animal things, like mating.
Sometimes we get curious to see what it is like to program computers
Dale Pendell, writing about the spirit of Salvia

Bruce Rimmell is not alone in his belief that Salvia (or, indeed, we) may have extraterrestrial origins. The scientist John Lilly and the psychologist Timothy Leary, after their own work with psychedelics (Ketamine and LSD, respectively) came to similar conclusions, while Terence McKenna believed that mushrooms arrived on our planet from another world as what he called 'Space spores'.

These scientists argued that if an advanced intelligence was trying to contact us it would do so not with messages from *outer* space but with communications to our *inner* space. As Karl Jansen explains in his book, *Ketamine: Dreams and Realities*: 'Like Lilly, Leary believed that extraterrestrial beings were more likely to contact us through inner rather than outer space on the basis that awareness can enter the inner quantum realm where the speed of light is transcended and non-local connections become possible.' The SETI (Search for Extraterrestrial Intelligence) project, which analyses radio signals from space in the search for other life is very old-tech after all, and very hit-or-miss since a message encoded in a burst of radio transmission, once passed our Earth and the range in which we can receive it, is gone until the next burst, and it may be a thousand years between signals. It is faster, simpler and more obvious and elegant, in a quantum universe, to communicate directly with the organism you wish to reach, consciousness-to-consciousness.

The idea is given credence not just by those scientists who have discovered a hidden code within the fabric of the universe, but by others who have found a similar code in our DNA.

According to authors Christopher Knight and Alan Butler,[7] 'When a team of genomic researchers [led by Edward Rubin] at the Lawrence Berkley National Laboratory in California presented their findings in June 2004, the audience [of fellow scientists] gasped in unison. Those listening simply could not believe what they were hearing.'

What Rubin and his team had discovered is that large sections of DNA could be removed from laboratory test subjects (mice) without any damage to them at all, including so-called 'conserved regions' of DNA. It is this which caused the surprise since conserved regions are highly protected areas thought to be vital to our survival. In Rubin's findings, however, these conserved regions could be removed without a problem because they were essentially protecting nothing, just areas of 'junk DNA'. The question was why, since, in the words of Knight and Butler, this protection is 'like having the world's finest encrypted security system built into your waste bin.'

Non-coded DNA – known as 'junk' – has traditionally been dismissed by scientists as useless since they could find no purpose for it, even though it comprises 97 percent of all life, including 97 percent of us. For it to have conserved regions seemed pointless – unless there was something going on in there that had been missed.

Knight and Butler continue: 'Any burglar who observed that your rubbish had so much apparently unnecessary protection would immediately suspect that you were hiding something of great value in an unexpected place. And that is the thought that occurred to [scientist] Paul Davies. He believes there could be a message from extra terrestrials in what has been referred to as junk DNA...' Another bizarre idea from the world of science and, again, one that is not without precedent.

'The feeling,' says Boston University physicist Eugene Stanley, 'is that there's something going on in the non-coding region.' Physicists noticed a few years ago, for example, that there are patterns in junk DNA: long-range correlations called 1/f noise, which suggested that it might contain some kind of organized information or message. Theorising that it might be a form of language, Stanley and his colleagues borrowed from the work of linguist George Zipf who had previously carried out a study of many hundreds of different texts to rank the frequency with which words occur. There is a distinct relationship pattern (now called Zipf's Law) which states that for any text in any language from any era the most frequently used word will occur twice as often as the second most frequent, which occurs twice as often as the fourth most frequent, and so on. In any text, that is – including the one you're holding – if the most frequently used word is 'the' and it appears 10,000 times, the next most common (e.g. 'and') will be used 5,000 times. The Law was developed and successfully used for code-breaking in espionage and war scenarios. Stanley applied it to DNA, testing it on 40 species ranging from viruses to humans. In every case, junk DNA followed Zipf's Law.

Every language also has built-in 'redundancies' so that a few confused words or typos do not make a sentence incomprehensible. We fill in the blanks and correct the mistakes ourselves so we still understand it. Knowing this, the researchers applied a second analysis; this one based on the work of information theorist Claude Shanon who in the 1950s had quantified redundancies in languages. They found that junk DNA contains nearly four times the redundancies of coding segments and follows a 'hierarchical arrangement of information'.

The simplest way to summarise this is to say that 97 percent of us (and of everything else) is not junk. It is language. Which begs the questions: Who put it there, why, and what does it say?

If we now add this new information to what we already know from quantum physicists – that we are living in a computer simulation – the conclusion seems clear: that junk DNA is the repository of a code that makes us act as we do within the programme of our posthuman descendents or the non-terrestrial entities which created us. It is what makes us a part of their matrix.

The reason that this is relevant to a book on Salvia is that this is exactly where the plant leads us too: to precisely these same conclusions. In this chapter I present trip reports from people around the world which demonstrate the point. Some of these people have worked with me in my Salvia research and workshops and some have conducted their own experiments and written their own accounts.[8] Bear in mind that the experience of working with salvinorin in particular, and the insights it gives us, can be so shocking that without a period of time to process what we have seen, the immediate feeling is often one of disorientation, and this is also evident in many of these accounts. With time to process, however, and with proper shamanic guidance, the fear and drama is lessened and reports like these generally become less incendiary, although the facts of the matter do not change.

What is interesting is how frequently the same sorts of images occur and, indeed, how often the same type of language is used by people who have in most cases never met or heard the accounts of their fellows. The themes that emerge are consistently ones of alienation, alien abduction, of being part of an experiment which is unknown, unknowable and far bigger than us, of other universes and other dimensions. Science is the art of making conclusions from evidence. Nothing may be real and nothing may ever be provable, but when the weight of evidence mounts we should at least pay attention to it.

Ultimately, as well, even though some of the themes seem

dark or negative (abduction and alienation etc), the conclusion is often hopeful and positive for those who take the journey. The point being that what these visionary motifs – and immersion in the Salvia experience itself – prove to us beyond doubt is that *nothing is real* in the way, at least, that we have been taught to see reality. And if that is the case, then those parts of us that have become central to our own stories and the myths we have of ourselves but which do not serve us well (for example, a belief that we are not worthy, not good enough, sick, damaged or that 'good things never happen to me') are equally false; illusions we have chosen to live by that we can now let go of and move on from in the knowledge that they also have no real meaning. Indeed, they may never have happened at all.

Dennis McKenna (himself no stranger to teacher plants, although I don't know about Salvia) writes about this in his book, *The Brotherhood of the Screaming Abyss*, commenting that, 'Among the most curious of my earliest remembrances are those that may not be real.' He goes on to describe an event from his early childhood where his older brother, Terence, pushed him down a flight of stairs. 'It's certainly a traumatic memory,' he continues, 'but did it really happen? I have no idea. Maybe it happened to someone else and I falsely remembered the experience as mine. Or perhaps I dreamt it… I continue to be astonished by how readily the mind confabulates, creating its own story to fill in the holes in memory, to the point where I can imagine looking back at the end of life and wondering if any of it really happened.'

As the psychologist Carl Jung put it: 'I am not what happened to me, I am what I choose to become'; words that Henry Thoreau would agree with, for, as the poet wrote: 'It's not what you look at that matters, it's what you *see*.' This is how Salvia heals: by giving us a new perspective on reality and on ourselves, even though the journey to get there can be a wild ride at times.

Ross and Deidre
(A personal account from original research conducted in Peru in 2010)

Having smoked, a street scene appeared; utterly real – like a wall or a wave of a different reality that moved through the room towards me. As it reached me I felt its particles pass through me like pins and needles and I realized that I could move around and through it. When I stepped into it I was in the street, when I stepped back I was in the room watching the reality wave approaching.

I asked my companion, Deidre, if she could see what I was seeing. It seemed so real that I couldn't imagine why she wouldn't – and in fact, she said she could. She saw blurred outlines of people – ghosts in the room – and me with my arm around someone as I surfed the reality-wave and walked with the people in the street. I took her hand and she felt solid, cold, meat-like, architectural even, while the others [those in the street] felt ethereal and tingly, like energy vibrations (and so did I when I was in their reality). I had a sense that even in everyday life other dimensions are always passing through us.

Deidre smoked next and found herself in the body of a machine in an alien factory, like a giant multi-levelled mangle, each layer a different scene – a beach, stars, country fields, a wall, standing stones – each of which was a vast self-contained world which she was a part of, like rolls of living wallpaper. A blue humanoid alien creature turned a handle and each of these worlds rolled forward until it folded in on itself. The people in these worlds panicked and ran as their reality slipped into the mangle and ended. The creature controlling it was amused at their reactions, their fear of annihilation, as if they/we really should have evolved beyond *that*.

Our 'reality' is actually multiple realities, and it is all just a play, maybe literally rolls of wallpaper each with a pattern, which contains its own consciousness, and is controlled by something bigger than us (the blue creature), which we might, I suppose, in our ignorance call 'God' and project all sorts of illusions onto but which is actually ambivalent, uninterested, and just a functionary in a factory. The world – or these multiple worlds around us – means very little in the whole scheme of things, nor does God or the factory-world he occupies because 'He' and we are all just cogs in a wheel.

Ross and Deidre
(Another account from original research conducted in Peru in 2010)

I smoked again and was back in the same street but something was different this time, and not quite right. The people were all dressed as if from the 1950s, the men in hats, tan suits, and brown brogues; the women in flared knee-high dresses, again in beige or tan – a limited palette although all of the colours were bright and pastel-like. Its just-so perfection was too nicely engineered, however, and the people too pink, as if they were drawings, cartoons coloured in by a child or a computer badly programmed to replicate skin tones but doing it just well enough to fool most of us most of the time.

It felt like an engineered world and I was now seeing beneath it. I could completely understand how conspiracy theorists like David Icke might conclude that the world is manipulated by powers we cannot comprehend but to name these powers as 'Illuminati' and pretend to know who (or what) they are was woefully simplistic of him. The truth of Salvia is even more disturbing: that we are nothing more than characters in a computer game perhaps played by an insignificant kid who really doesn't care about us at all. At least in Icke's cosier view of things those who seek to control us can be located in time and space and care enough about us to bother with their manipulations of our reality. What we learn from Salvia, however, is that we have no idea who is 'playing' us – and that there is more to reality than Icke's Illuminati, who, by definition, exist in a universe that can at least be comprehended if not seen. The comprehensible universe, however, is merely a footnote, if that, to what Salvia knows. Whatever that is, we can also be sure that, like any kid with a toy, we are no more important or significant to those who ultimately own us than the next distraction which comes along.

As my journey continued, I found myself in another street, this time with no people, just an empty road with houses on each side, something like the street I grew up in. I *knew*, however, that this was just a film, a projection onto fabric, and it felt like this is what all reality is: a projection we make onto fabric. I began to physically tear the screen apart; I wanted to know what is on the other side. But there was nothing, only blackness. I entered it and began to drift through the emptiness of space. Looking back I could see that Earth/the reality I've just left is a cube and there are other cubes/planets/realities all around me. Within each of them is a multiverse and I realize just how vast and intricate and wholly mysterious what we call 'reality' is. The cubes also looked like the hexagonal patterns that Salvia produces when it is smoked and perhaps, I thought, Salvia itself contains these realities; that it is a plant which enables us not just to explore multiple worlds (like ayahuasca) or to more fully experience this world (like San Pedro), but which gives us access to completely other dimensions.

'Possibility number one,' writes Dennis McKenna in *The Brotherhood of the Screaming Abyss*, 'is that there actually are other dimensions, parallel realities that these substances [like Salvia] render accessible by temporarily altering our neurochemistry and perceptual apparatus. According to this model, there really are entities that want to communicate with us, or at least don't spurn communication when we poke our heads into their dimension. This is very close to the understanding of reality that prevails in most shamanic worldviews.

'The conclusions… are rather earth-shattering… [since] we are forced to reject or at least radically revise everything we think we know about reality. It makes our current models hopelessly obsolete and incomplete. All of human knowledge, all of science and religion, must be re-examined in the light of the understanding that our cosmic neighbourhood just 'over there' is of a completely different ontological order and, moreover, an order that is inhabited by entities as intelligent as we are, or many times more intelligent, but that share with us the quality of consciousness, of mindedness. And they are entities that want to share their reality with us, their wisdom, their knowledge, perhaps even form a symbiotic partnership or some form of diplomatic relationship. Whatever 'they' are, they do not seem to be hostile, and they appear to take a compassionate interest in our species, much as an adult might want to love and nurture a child.'

It is a 'compassionate interest' delivered by a cold and dispassionate species, however, and sometimes more than the human soul or mind can bear. Despite our propensity for conflict and violence, for example, we are still able to feel love and warmth. But then, perhaps that may also be our problem: too much 'heat' and not enough clinical distance. Our alien neighbours can certainly teach us that.

Somatzu
(From accounts at Erowid.org)

Everything around me was very alien. I looked at Joe; he was standing behind the camera [videoing the session] and he let out a couple of laughs. This had a terrible effect on me and constituted the hardest part of the trip; I now thought Joe was some alien being who videotaped all of human existence for his own pleasure and he was laughing at how ridiculous this silly little human was. I totally freaked out and curled up wondering if he would kill me or keep me alive in his dimension.

... I felt a deep terror that still haunts me when I think about it. I started screaming for help...

Trendal
(An account at Erowid.org)

Suddenly I became aware of a series of strange zipper-like patterns across the room, running parallel with the floor... Then I noticed the presence of a few beings around me whom I thought to be my friends... Each of these beings was attached to one of the zipper lines in some way I can't describe... The idea was passed to me from somewhere that these people were the heads of the zippers that held reality together. This was, I assure you, one of the most intricate horrors I have ever come across. The idea that these people were all that stood between reality and nothingness scared the living shit out of me.

To my complete horror I watched as one of my former friends began to walk along his zipper-line with an insane grin on his face. Reality began to 'unzip'. I don't know how else to describe it. It looked *exactly* like a zipper being undone. The two sections of reality that were previously joined by the zipper began to spread apart. An infinite blackness was the only thing left between the sheets of reality.

My friends, I realized, were only some benevolent consciousness wearing their skin. Each one moved and acted precisely the same way. Each with the same sick grin on his face, they would unzip their zipper while goading me into letting it happen... I realized that I had no control over the situation and never had.

The beings wearing my friends' faces changed from goading and sneaky to angry and forceful. I was chased out of my room, into the kitchen. I became aware of the fact that I could not move as I thought I should be able to. There was some form of resistance whenever I moved, accompanied by a strange zipping sound. I was now a zipper head and as I ran I was unzipping reality behind me.

Panic hit me very, very fast. I tried to flee the kitchen as the other zippers had followed me and were trying to catch up to me for what I thought was some purely evil reason. It was imperative that I stay ahead of them if I were to survive. I made my way through the living room, down the back hallway of my house, out the back door. Reality was now completely coming apart around me. Everything had gone quiet except for the noise of the other zippers following me and the noise my own zipper made as I moved. All other noise seemed to disappear as reality was unzipped. I was now in a very real state of panic as I watched in horror as my house unzipped from reality. I was not safe outside either, I realized.

DoOr
(An account at Erowid.org)

I saw/felt... my Self being completely and quite literally unzipped. I saw the fucking teeth of the zipper separating.

Glassalchemist
(An account at Erowid.org)

Where am I? How did I get here? What is the meaning of this? Immediately, a voice jumps into my thoughts, explaining that this is where you go when you fall asleep. All of the races go there. Together in their slumber, their thoughts intertwine and intermingle to form the web I would best understand as the multiverses. The voice explained that our collective consciousness is what keeps the multiverse in existence. It was horrible. We are enslaved in our sleep, harvested to allow this gargantuan machine... to pump all of our energy around at high speeds...

This place [planet Earth] is so strange. So pointless... I hope one day we will all wake up and smash that fucking dream machine. It is a trap. It is there to enslave our energy. We should be in control of our own souls, our own destiny.

MacExistence
(An account at Erowid.org)

All around... was a giant empty void, not really black, just sort of no-thing. I totally felt as if my body was this giant void... Then after what seemed like near eternity... the perception of my body went from being that huge void to being trapped in a small container about the size of my head, which was very confusing and confining, as if I was forced in it.

Vulpine
(An account at Erowid.org)

I was a five-pointed wheel. Reality itself was the five-spoked wheel... It had infinite depth, like each spoke of the wheel was a long shelf stretching out into the distance. It was kind of like a paddle wheel on a boat, only each of the five buckets was infinitely long and deep. I was actually a consciousness inside the tumbling object, rotating in its chambers while aware of all the chambers. They were full of light and beautifully riotous colours.

As I tumbled in my colourful bucket, through an opening in my chamber, I could sometimes see out into another world, the base or real reality... I became cognizant that my entire life, or what I had perceived it to be, all twenty-seven years, were actually an illusion. They were merely a fancy I had generated while watching the interplay of light, colour and shadow in my bucket. Any minute now I would be tumbled out onto the grass, forever lost from this false, comfortable reality and loosed into the base reality outside, forever cut off from the illusion of my life I was used to.

Similar themes

It is worth contrasting that account with Lela's, later on in this book, who also connects the symbol of the wheel to a sort of karmic cycle of life before and beyond death, a sort of 'viewing station' between incarnations and worlds, and the following account from Kira Salak, which appeared in National Geographic magazine. Hers was an experience arising from ayahuasca rather than Salvia, but the themes are very similar.

Now I'm travelling to a realm where I meet my various incarnations from past lives. We are connected to a large wheel; whenever fear energy leaves the top of my head in puffs of dark smoke, it leaves their heads at the same time. Our lives, it seems, are interconnected and dependent. Outside of linear time, all our lifetimes, all our many incarnations, occur simultaneously. 'Past life' is really a misnomer; 'other life' seems a more accurate way of describing it.

With some of the individuals [in my vision], I can guess their historical period from their clothing. With others, I can't place them at all. There is a balding, overweight, monk-looking guy. The big muscular warrior with the pointed helmet (who, he says, gives me my present interest in the martial arts). The black woman who is a slave in North Carolina. Interestingly, there are only about 15 or so individuals; a spirit tells me that many people average less than 30 total Earth incarnations and that their souls commonly skip centuries, reincarnating only in spirit realms. And what of the two women who aren't wearing historically identifiable clothing? 'We are your future incarnations,' one of them explains, lovingly.[9]

John
(A client who joined me for a private healing retreat to work with Salvia)

I could feel the floor beneath me spinning and carrying me around the outer edge of a wheel that now filled the room, and it felt like chaos. It was only when I remembered what I was doing here that I found myself at the centre of the spinning, then it felt like the entire universe was moving around me. Somebody said, 'You've been here before.' I didn't feel any personality to Salvia except something metallic not flesh. There was a paradox beneath it all: like pure mathematics with an organic feel, like everything could be angular and circular at the same time.

[In my vision] I was watching a TV show about plants from outer space. Then suddenly I was in the show and the whole thing opened up interdimensionally... It felt like there is something really big, something we don't understand that is controlling things in a way we can't know. A real existential terror... I always had a fear of alien abduction, of being taken against my will and being out of control and [it] felt like that...

The reality I was in became a pulsing fragment of something larger – real, unreal, surreal. I found myself – if I *was* a self – asking, Where am I? Who am I? What should I do? *Reality is alive*: in a physical yet mechanical way! I realized that I am just part of it, and I can't separate myself from anything else. At one point I opened my eyes and looked at you but I had no idea who you were or who I was.

When I started to come round a little I saw this huge machine and all of these people were walking out of it. They were all identical, clean and dressed in white clothes. It felt like a rebirthing machine, like the people coming out of it had been washed clean in it so they were new and hadn't had any ideas or beliefs forced onto them or any experiences that had shaped them. There were no patterns.

[That night] I had dreams about authority and freedom. In the first we were living in a police state but it was also like a school we were put in against our will. Some of us created a plot to get out where we dressed as police officers and stole a car but even outside the compound, authority was everywhere and they found us and sent us back. It wasn't a horrible place but it was a prison and the guards thought it important for us to be there because that was their dream. In another I was aboard a spacecraft with lots of other people, like a kind of ark, but the engine died and we couldn't take off. Again we were boarded by police who said we couldn't leave and searched us for drugs. We could never get where we wanted.

Marla
(A student who smoked Salvia as part of my Plant Spirit Wisdom workshop)

We were all lying down in a perfect line like seeds or cocoons on a spaceship and the room was divided into squares by bright lights. It felt like déjà vu because I have seen this somewhere before. The whole thing felt metallic. It was like we were being used in some way or I was in an experiment… like we were all on the same mission… a dream within a dream.

The important thing for me is that I didn't want to be a seed because I saw it as programmed, like it was made for someone else's use, so they could plant it and get what they wanted. The seed represented potential and I wanted it for myself.

Crystallinesheen
(An account at Erowid.org)

You know when a person gets to that point past that little crust of perception that we call 'Our Lives' and 'Our World?' Where they suddenly realize their ultimate position in life and the universe? It's not fun as it totally invalidates our lives. I mean, when you realize that everybody you love and everything you take for granted about 'this world' are merely props on an intergalactic stage? All of our hopes, dreams, fears, just soap bubbles on the plate of existence? I mean, we all know that we are merely shells walking around on this earth but when you actually SEE that, oh god, it SUCKS, SUCKS, SUCKS. Some things we aren't meant to see while we are still bound in meat reality…

At least on acid that time in New Orleans, experiencing a similar vision, I knew that when the acid faded I could return to the comfortable delusion that is (was?) my life... It wasn't like that on Salvia. I was watching the credits roll on my entire life. Even if I survived what did it matter? You can't have infinity and humanity at the same time, they don't work well together.

Rob
(A student who smoked Salvia as part of my Plant Spirit Wisdom workshop)

Within seconds of smoking, Rob began to make loud noises: slurred, unrecognizable words, screams, groans, roars, and deep vocal sounds, which at times had the feel of an alien language. Those close to him who had also smoked said they could understand it and among what he said was, 'Stop laughing at me.' To those of us who had not taken Salvia it sounded like glossolalia: speaking in tongues. He began thrashing, flailing his arms and legs and rolling backward and forward. After some minutes he got up and staggered to the door. I followed him out and he stood in the night air, holding his head and muttering, 'Oh fuck, fuck. What is this? What's happening to me?' He needed to be outside for the rest of the ceremony but calmed down and returned to normalcy after about 50 minutes. Later, he provided this account:

I was immediately folded up into nothing. Then a sort of digital structure began shaping me, replicating me out of existence until I became everything and nothing. I felt extreme anxiety and this increased the process of the replication to warp speed. The last piece of me was now vanishing into digital information and I started fighting it and trying to put myself back together but I was panicking. Someone came over to help me but even his hand on my arm felt alien. There was no 'me' now and the 'reality' around me, both inside the room and wherever I was, was chaos. I heard laughter and thought I was the butt of everyone's joke. I couldn't speak and felt stupid and alone, with no friends and unworthy of love: a very raw feeling.

When I settled down I asked Salvia what I should make of all this and she told me that all of my fears had attached themselves to me over many years until I had become small in the face of everyone else's ideas. Fear had tried to cheat me into a denial of myself but Salvia said I was rare and special and that I can choose love over fear any time I want because even a personality based on fear can be loved, and once fear leaves love becomes unconditional.

After the ceremony finished I revisited Salvia [in my mind] and she explained that I had time travelled. I had gone back in time and attached myself to certain situations where power had been taken from me through fear and I had become spread out very thinly into bits of me.

I hadn't been able to sleep at all, and now I heard a cock crow and saw the light of the dawn. Salvia said we are all capable of time travel. I looked around and it had become dark and the cock crowed again *for the first time.*

I had *actually* travelled in time, from the light of dawn back into darkness and then the dawn again. Salvia said she wanted to demonstrate how easy time travel was. She said that all human beings are capable of time travel – literally – but we are not ready for it yet. We need to walk before we can run or we will fragment as I had and become attached to other existences, then we will be lost in a nightmare. We have started to learn the process of time travel because some of us now realize that what we believe to be true *makes* it true. This is step one.

Throughout the experience I was as scared as shit but I feel it had a happy ending and I learned a lot about myself and what is really real.

Rob did not know this because participants on my workshops

have no access to internet, newspapers or TV but just two days before his Salvia journey the CERN atomic research facility in Geneva had announced its discovery of particles that can move faster than light (so-called 'God Particles'), disproving Einstein's theorem E=MC2, which has become a cornerstone of modern scientific theory and which relies on the 'fact' that nothing can exceed light speed. That is no longer true (obviously, in fact, it never was).

One implication of this is that time travel, as Salvia had said, must (theoretically at least) be possible since it is already, in effect, taking place at a sub-atomic level. The particles that CERN explores are the same ones that we are made of, of course, which also suggests that time travel is possible from within us, again as Salvia had said.

Salvia Teachings

These accounts give a flavour of what Salvia is here to teach us. From them and many others, I provided a checklist in my books *Shamanic Quest for the Spirit of Salvia* and *Drinking the Four Winds* of the common themes that tend to emerge during Salvia journeys. These are some of them:

Personal Identity

The questions 'Who am I?' and 'Who are you?' are frequently raised, as some of the examples above also show. We tend to take our identity and our history for granted, accepting it as a given that the things we 'know' about ourselves are real. But are they? Most of us can summarise our lives in a matter of minutes, for example, but, by definition, what we are giving is a life *story*, a synopsis, invention and dramatisation since a real history would take as long to relate, second-by-second, as the age you are now.

And even then it wouldn't be reliable since, according to psychologists, our brain 'creates the *illusion* of a detailed perception but at the same time discards details which it considers to be irrelevant – even if these details are decidedly out of the ordinary. American psychologists Christopher Chabris and Daniel Simons showed Harvard University students a short video clip of people playing basketball. The students were asked to count the number of passes made by the team wearing white. Almost every participant got the correct answer but half completely missed the man in a gorilla suit who walks across the screen during the video. *Inattentional blindness* is the name given to [this], our brain's limited receptiveness.'[10]

Similarly, if we are determined or conditioned to view ourselves in a particular way, this is how we present ourselves in our life stories – as victims or heroes or villains, for example – ignoring evidence to the contrary (the men in gorilla suits) which does not fit our script. The philosopher Ram Dass put it simply: 'What, after all, is personal history if not a dream?' And we can make that dream be whatever we want.

In fact, what Salvia shows us is that we are actually *nothing at all*. As Siebert remarked after his initial journey with salvinorin: 'I had no *actual* memory of ever having lived'; a comment similar to that made earlier by Dennis McKenna, and by Blosser after his experiences with Salvia: 'I was not aware that I… had ever [even] had a body.'

Rob, in my own research, (see above) says much the same thing: 'There was no 'me'.' In his account we see again the panic that this realisation can cause – but because of it there is also healing and hope. If, after all, we are literally nothing, just characters in a game or an experiment conducted by others then, at least as far as our perception of ourselves goes, we can choose *any* life story, identity or outcome we wish. We do not *have* to be the villain or the victim every time. We do not *have* to be ill. We do not *have* to be the drug addict, the sex addict, the gambler or the drunk, even if it is a role that is familiar to us and one that others readily cast us into. We *can* change. It may take an act of will but we can do it because *we* are not our *stories*.

As the novelist Chuck Palahniuk wrote in his book *Fight Club*, 'You are not your job. You're not how much money you have in the bank. You are not the car you drive. You're not the contents of your wallet. You are not your fucking khakis.' We may still be the 'all-singing, all-dancing crap of the world' in a simulation created by others but we are also powerful and unique. This is the paradox that Salvia also reveals. In quantum reality, after all, 'the opposite of one profound truth may very well be another profound truth,' as the physicist Niels Bohr remarked.

Bobby, another participant on my *Plant Spirit Wisdom* workshop put it in her own way when she said that '[With Salvia] all boundaries were gone and it seemed possible to be or do anything... boundary-less participation in the mind of the universe was ecstatic.' It doesn't have to be a nightmare to realise that while we are the plaything of the 'gods'; we are also free. Or as free as we *want* to be, at least.

Parallel Universes and Other Dimensions

I have speculated in other books about the interdimensionality of Salvia: that it is capable of taking us to a place outside time and space and linking us to something greater than both – the awareness, in quantum terms, that there is no time or space (since computer code is immaterial).

Another of my participants referred to the 'interdimensional gateways' opened up by the plant. Others, like Trendal and DoOr in the accounts above, see reality as being 'unzipped' and whatever lies behind it coming through.

The quantum physicist Michio Kaku has remarked that, 'We [scientists] are forced to confront the idea of other dimensions. It is the only theory that has been able to unify all the laws of physics.' These dimensions are in fact all around us at all times although we do not notice them, just as radio waves and microwaves and cosmic radiation are all around us unseen. It takes a change in perspective – a new way of seeing or a piece of equipment capable of sensing what we cannot – for them to be revealed. For the shaman, Salvia is this equipment and through it new dimensions are opened.

Time Travel

Since essentially there is no time, 'time travel' should, paradoxically, be easy. Of course, we would not be travelling to other periods (since that would be illogical: there *is* no time) but into an awareness of experiences that have happened or have yet to happen to us – what we might nominally call 'the past' or 'the future', although in reality (that is, in shamanic and quantum reality) these timeframes do not actually exist because everything is taking place in the Infinite Now.

Siebert, in his first experiment with salvinorin, refers to an experience of this kind; of 'revisiting places from childhood', such as his grandparents' living room furnished as it was when he was a child. 'This *was* the real world,' he says, 'not a memory or a vision. I was *really* there and it was all just as solid as the room I'm sitting in now... All the points of time in my personal history coexisted. One did not precede the next. Apparently, had I so willed it, I could return to any point in my life and *really be there* because it was actually happening right *now*.'

During my first journeys with Salvia I was also taken back to my childhood and found myself with my mother in a street I knew 40 years ago. These were not memories either because the events that took place in my visions were not recollections of things I know to have happened or significant enough to have been 'issues' that I have repressed. To me, as for Seibert, they were entirely real and happening in the moment when I (re-)experienced them. Salvia was giving me an opportunity to revisit the 'past' and not exactly relive it but change my view of it (and consequently change the future and present as well) by experiencing it in a new way that also had a new impact now. In other words, these were not memories but a form of time travel:

dimensional shifts to a place where the paths of the universe had bifurcated because of a decision I had made then, and now I was able to take another of its paths simply by making a new choice to perceive the events of my childhood differently, experiencing them again from a new perspective.

J D Arthur, in his book, *Salvia Divinorum*, has a similar idea. 'If, as science tells us,' he remarks, 'time itself can be altered by unrelated factors such as gravity and motion perhaps other factors of a more penetrating interior nature should not be dismissed... ironically, time itself, it seems, needs a perceiver of its passage to exist.'

This form of time travel offers us another possibility for life and for healing. Many of us, I suppose, have had difficult childhood moments which, consciously or otherwise, we carry around with us as part of our life *stories*, defining ourselves in terms of a judgement or an event that happened years ago; still living it, in effect, and acting it out when the moment itself has long passed.

It is often the subtlest things which have the greatest impact on us. A female client once told me, for example, how she had lost her virginity at the age of fourteen. She planned it and deliberately set out to entice the man she wanted but the act, when it happened, was more like rape than a loving encounter. She didn't mention it to anybody but wrote about it in her diary, later discovering that her intrusive and controlling father had read through it and against that entry had written the single word 'slut'.

Almost in defiance of her father, she quickly set out on a quest for independence through parties, drugs and sex. By her early 30s she couldn't remember how many men and women she had slept with, but well in excess of 50, sometimes with more than one at once. It took her years to realise that it was not the 'rape' which had traumatised her but her father's *judgement of her* and that, rather than freedom, she had for much of her life been imprisoned by a word. Because of it she became the embodiment of his judgement, a cliché of a self-fulfilling prophecy, sleeping with anyone, strangers and friends alike, as the mood took her in her 'quest for freedom'. Perhaps she had set out unconsciously to punish her father or prove him wrong about her but she became the very thing he saw her as and, ironically, the person she hurt most was herself, some of the consequences of her actions being a string of abortions and a case of cervical cancer.

Another woman had never wanted children because her own childhood had been difficult, especially with her father who had caused her so much pain and distress that she had become addicted to drugs and alcohol as a way of escaping from him and from life. Her decision not to have children was at least partly motivated by her desire to hurt the father who had hurt her. 'I didn't want to make him a grandfather so he could damage somebody else's life,' she said. But by doing so, however, she also damaged herself. Her father died when she was 50 and by then it was too late for her to conceive. It was at that point that she realised she would have loved a child of her own and, through her son or daughter, might also have healed the wounds of her past.

A final example is Doris, who I knew through a business venture in Spain where we opened a healing centre together. Although it had been a long-time dream of hers to do so, almost from the start Doris had little to do with the centre and left Spain altogether just a year or so into our partnership. Her departure was motivated, she said, because her daughters were having children of their own and she wanted to be back in England with them. But that is not the whole truth. I knew from what she had told me that her marriage had been difficult and motherhood had been hard for her and that she felt guilty for what she had put her children through. That was the deeper cause for what became a doting obsession with her family now. Her return from Spain (and her guilt) cost Doris her business, her dream and, eventually, almost £100,000 of her life savings and her children's inheritance when the centre she gave up was sold at a loss.

At the level of the soul, dramas like these consume us or, in the computer language we have been using in this book, they become part of our programming. But what if we could revisit the events of our lives which caused them and re-experience them from a position of adult power instead of the powerlessness and fears of a wounded child? Then we might be able to change them and take back what we lost of ourselves. By offering us its peculiar access to time travel Salvia gives us the therapeutic potential to do that. One of my students, Darryl, summarised his own experiences in this way: 'The Shepherdess [Salvia] helps me to see all that may ever be' – and not just the limited reality that we are habituated into.

> *Humans too are unfinished... As Jean-Paul Sartre said, we are our own projects: we are what we shall become, and what we shall become is a matter of our choices. We want to grow, to achieve, to find, to discover, to make, to produce, to reproduce – in short, we seek those activities in life that matter to us. So although we are unfinished and incomplete, we are progressive beings. We never achieve finality but we are always becoming something more*
> David Suits[11]

A greater array of choices and other universes to explore means a greater possibility of becoming something other than we are.

Being Out of Body

Being out of body with Salvia is nothing like lucid dreaming, 'core shamanic' journeying or 'gently floating above oneself', as the new age literature sometimes describes the out-of-body state. Rather, it is like being catapulted out of the self and any awareness of corporeal being. As Blosser remarked: 'I was not aware that I… had ever *had* a body.'

The process of getting out of the self with Salvia can be a rough ride; immediate, jarring, and with a sensation that some describe as being ripped apart, unzipped, dismembered or dismantled. The journey does not happen just on a spiritual or emotional level or in terms of 'awareness' but *physically*. One of my participants, Sue, recalls how her body was 'pulled backward, twisted and contorted' – a common experience at the onset of Salvia – while another, Lela, felt herself 'flying over the room'. At the same time, she was not actually aware that she had – or had ever had – a 'self'.

J D Arthur writes about his own experiences as containing a 'seemingly very real potential for leaving the body', which to him felt 'remarkably natural... In the months to come this sensation – that I could abandon the normal physical matrix almost at will – became a regular feature… and seems to be the mechanism of many of the transformative processes that have made their appearance over the course of time.' It is worth noting, however, that Arthur usually worked with 5X Salvia extracts (i.e. at the lower end of the scale) and so describes a far gentler journey than most. At concentrates of 100X, 50X or even 20X, the sensation of leaving the body can be anything but gentle. Others have described it as like 'being in a wind tunnel', 'being pulled rapidly backward through space' or 'having the skin ripped from my back'.[12]

In shamanic terms we would say that Salvia aids the ability to journey by assisting the soul to take flight from the body. Unlike the 'core shamanic' (if there is such a thing) journey, however, there is no control over the flight of the soul or its destination during the initial 'blast-off' stages when Salvia is smoked, and only limited control during the rest of the journey, especially at higher doses, even after considerable experience and training. Those who practice core shamanism therefore and believe that this is what 'shamanism' is should take especial note that

working with Salvia is very real, not an imaginative psychospir-
itual process, and will therefore be nothing like what they are
used to. Indeed, part of the function of the plant is to remove the
'psychology' from the 'self' so we enter the 'spirit worlds' fully
and without the 'mind-stuff' – the artifice and analysing –
common to modern Western shamanic techniques.

Intention

Since all shamanic work has a point and a purpose (it is never
just about 'tripping'), intention is still key (whether to gather
information, reveal possible futures, or seek healing). The
problem, though, is that you are unlikely to be able to hold on to
this intention as the sage takes grip. Again, 'core shamans' please
take note.

The best solution to this is a three-stage process where:

1. The intention is held while smoking or chewing the
   leaves, then
2. Forgotten or ignored as the plant provides answers
   through the journey (since trying to hold on to an
   intention is a losing battle and will interfere with the
   process anyway), then, finally to
3. Return to your intention during the 30 minutes or so of
   silence and contemplation that should follow a Salvia
   journey. In this dream state you will remember more of
   the journey and, by reference to your original intention,
   be able to make greater sense of the images and
   symbols you were shown.

It is also a good idea to have an observer or 'sitter' with you as
you journey so they can take care of you when your own physical
control is lost. You can then also compare notes when the session
has ended since you will almost certainly have missed or
forgotten part of your experience. As an example of both loss of

control and loss of memory, I once sat for a woman in Spain during a 100X extract session. As soon as the Salvia hit her she began babbling, speaking animatedly to someone in front of her who only she could see, rolling on the floor and throwing herself at a wall before finally lying on the ground unmoving for 20 minutes. Despite what appeared to me to be a great deal of content to her journey, she could remember none of it when she returned.[13]

Overlapping Realities

During the experience I wrote about earlier, when I found myself in a street from my childhood with my mother,[14] I observed at the time that, 'Every object in my life was also me; like our realities were interchangeable,' so I was able to experience reality (and see myself) from the perspective of all of the things and objects around me – even those as seemingly random and insignificant as a brick, a leaf or a bus stop. In fact, it is not enough to say that I *'experienced* reality' from *their* perspective; *I was those things*. All of them were conscious and aware and shared a purpose and intelligence with me, 'as if a sort of pre-birth agreement had been made between us that we would share this reality together,' each of us a part of the whole.

Others have experienced this too and merged consciousness during their journeys with a variety of non-human things, becoming wallpaper, a suitcase, a wardrobe, a brick, a zipper... It sounds ridiculous, but for those unused to it, losing all sense of ever being human and knowing absolutely that you are merely 'digital information', as my participant Roy put it, is anything but amusing. Try it sometime. Nor should those familiar with psychedelics and entheogens dismiss this as simply a form of 'ego death'. It is far more than that.

How it feels is much as the scientist J B S Haldane remarked, that, 'The universe is not only stranger than we imagine, it is stranger than we *can* imagine.' It can also be extremely unsettling when that universe, of its own volition, takes control of you and provides you with an experience which *exceeds* the powers of your imagination.

What Salvia is doing by giving us these experiences is showing us, graphically and directly once more that we are not human beings and never were. We are energy or code or information; the same energy that makes up everything that we perceive in our universe. Through this we are connected to all things at all times. We know them because *we are them* at the deepest energy levels. This connection also accounts for the empathetic, telepathic and precognitive states that Salvia gives access to (see below) and for its reputation as a plant of divination (future-seeing), since the future, along with the past and the present, exists only Now in a timeless universe.

Wheels within Wheels

The motifs of wheels and cogs appear commonly in Salvia journeys. My participants have found themselves part of 'circles that joined together' or 'trapped on a huge cog which was rotating, going round and round', or they may become 'a five-pointed wheel' themselves and discover that, 'Reality itself was the five-spoked wheel... It had infinite depth, like each spoke of the wheel was a long shelf stretching out into the distance.. . like a paddle wheel on a boat.'

The wheel or circle is a symbol that has been used across ages and cultures to signify wholeness, completion, unity, love, the circle of life or the wheel of destiny. It may also mean any of these things during a Salvia journey and act as a reminder from the plant about what is important in life: completion of ourselves through awareness of what is real (and unreal) about our lives, although its precise significance will also, for this very reason, be different for everyone who sees it.

Even so, the symbol often appears in relation to a need for love and completion. The first time she smoked, one of my participants, Deidre, felt 'a rolling sensation' and saw what she described as 'a huge waterwheel', accompanied by 'a sense of something from her childhood'. She was at the time dealing with family issues and dramas that went back to her preteen years and in particular with the toxic residue of a father who she described as emotionally and physically abusive and who she thought might also have had a sexual interest in her.

Another participant who joined a different ceremony to gain insight into repetitive and dysfunctional relationship patterns also saw himself as 'trapped... going around and around', as in fact Deidre was doing in her own way. As a final example, a female participant actually *became* a wheel during her ceremony[15] and began uncontrollably rolling in circles on the floor. The emotional issue she had come to deal with was the guilt she felt over the loss of her child. After the ceremony ended she was able to talk about this, and to begin her healing. 'I realized that circling [i.e. carrying such guilt forever and going over and over the same ground] is no fun. In the centre [of the circle]... I was whole again.'

Telepathy and Empathy

Feelings of connection, togetherness, empathy and even telepathy are mentioned by many Salvia smokers. My participant Michael commented after ceremony that, 'It was like I had telepathy because I thought I could hear [another participant] talking to me from across the room [and] just as I thought that she began to crawl over to me,' while another, Bobby, remarked that, '[Salvia] seemed to add to a sense of our togetherness and was a bit telepathic – I wasn't sure if we were speaking or sharing thoughts.'

Others have said the same thing while working independently with Salvia. Alexia is a psychotherapist in the UK, for example, and sometimes smokes the plant an hour or so before she sees clients. She says that, 'On many occasions when I have worked with clients [after smoking Salvia] I have been hyper-intuitive to their needs and issues and they have commented on this.' Once again, we are all the same energy (or, if you prefer, part of the same computer programme) so this sense of connection is unsurprising when we let go of the rational mind and stop pretending that we are separate and independent beings.

Coldness and Distance: The Personality of the Plant

David Suits writes in Philosophy Now (January 2002) that:

Two millennia ago the Stoic philosopher Epictetus pointed out that some things are under our complete control and some things are not, and if we try to control anything which is not under our control, then we are setting ourselves up for frustration, which is a kind of unhappiness. So in order to avoid unhappiness we ought to give up trying to control the uncontrollable. But which things are those?

The answer, for Epictetus, was simple: everything outside of your own thoughts is not completely under your control. What matters is *your attitude*. Epictetus recommended an emotional detachment from the world, which is accomplished only by accepting the world as it is [as it *truly* is], being satisfied with what actually happens and not railing against the gods for making the world be one way when you passionately wanted it to be otherwise. Give up those passions, they pave the road to frustration.

But it is hard to cultivate an untroubled mind because it requires considerable wisdom, strict reasoning and unbiased logic. Yet there is no higher serenity than being a spectator. To be a player is to gamble with happiness and to risk losing.

This Stoic philosophy is in some ways also Salvia philosophy.

The plant, as a teacher, would disagree with little that Epictetus believed; perhaps only that we have control over even our own thoughts, since we have already seen how perception, memory, our life *stories* and the impacts of others such as parents and lovers can produce drives in us which lead to unconscious and even self-destructive behaviours. However, we do have the *potential* to know ourselves better and so (in a sense) take charge of our lives, and plants like Salvia can help. Our attitude – our aware approach to life – is, indeed, key. But in turning to Salvia for insight, we should also know what we are getting into.

The 'new age' has cultivated a rather silly idea that the plants used by shamans are all loving, warm and friendly. Pretty little flowers. Working with them is at worst seen as a harmless endeavour that probably won't teach you much, but more usually they are regarded as charming servants, always happy to help, something like 'fairies' or 'angels'. As I am sure you must have gathered by now, however, there is nothing 'fluffy' about Salvia. My client John described her as, 'Like pure mathematics with an organic feel' – cold, clinical and no-nonsense. Dale Pendell, who has also written about this plant, says simply: 'Is there any more direct?'

Salvia simply tells it like it is. Straight to the point. Then you can either take it or leave it and cope with the truths she reveals or do your best to ignore or hide from them. In *Shamanic Quest for the Spirit of Salvia*, for example, I relate the story of how my wife decided, without warning or explanation, to leave our marriage one day. I thought she had gone crazy (or I had). Still, wanting to leave the door open for her in case she chose to return, I kept my wedding ring on and told her I would welcome her back if she promised to talk things over with me so we could deal with her issues. Her response was angry, abusive emails, but still no explanation, followed by silence.

Working with Salvia to try to understand what was going on, I asked the plant why this was happening, but it simply laughed at me for making her any offer at all in return for her promise to talk. 'She married you, didn't she?' the plant asked, bluntly. 'What more important promise could she make – and she couldn't even keep that!'

It was about as direct and unemotional as it could get, but I knew that the plant was right and took off my wedding ring. Strangely enough, a few hours later my wife phoned for the first and only time, although she had nothing worthwhile or important to say, just how much she loved and missed me and our life together in Spain – and how determined she was never to return. Salvia, a plant with a reputation for taking us beyond the bounds of sanity, made more sense than she did.

It had also delivered what I asked for, however – contact with my wife – and shown me how pointless it was. I chose the saner option from then on and left my wedding ring off. Then I moved on, following the blunt, but sound advice of the sage.

Freewill versus Determinism: 'It is what it is'

Are we free or are our actions determined? We make choices every hour of the day, of course – but are they truly *ours*? As we saw above, for example, our life histories, *stories*, experiences, joys and triumphs, sorrows and losses, the conditioning which began in us even before we were born – in our mother's womb, in our parents' genes – have all led us to this one singular moment of choice and although *we* make it our entire ancestral line stands behind us watching our every move. So is it really *our* choice?

Within the bigger picture, if we are part of a programme or characters in a game, is it we who act or does someone act for us? And even if the latter, but we believe it *our* choice, then, in a way, is it still?

Many novelists say that when they write books, for example, their characters 'take on a life of their own'. They are still characters and operate within the plot laid out by the writer but they also have an influence on their creator. They become his life too, so who is really writing who?

This is not just an intellectual exercise. It has implications which Salvia wants us to see. My client Sahara's personal history, for example – the experiences she told me about experiencing at the hands of her parents and the way she was bullied at school – made it pretty obvious why personal relationships were difficult for her, why trust and vulnerability were issues she struggles with, and why she has a tendency to run from intense emotions. All of these factors made it quite inevitable that she would one day leave someone she loved to impress the father she hated – and yet it was still *she* who chose to act that way. And she is not unique: we all have relationships (first and foremost, with ourselves) and similar influences act upon us.

This issue – freewill versus determinism and the contradictions it seems to pose – is one which has concerned many philosophers. 'Some believe that humans have free will; others that each of our actions and choices is caused by prior events. *Compatibilism* is the theory that we can be both caused and free,' writes Craig Ross in Philosophy Now (August 2007).

'Hobbes famously wrote that man was as free as an unimpeded river. A river that flows down a hill necessarily follows a channel but it is also at liberty to flow within the channel. The voluntary actions of people are similar. They are free because their actions follow from their will but their actions are also necessary because they spring from chains of causes and effects which could in principle be traced back to the first mover of the universe, generally called God.'

What are some of the implications for this in our lives? Well, suppose you love your parents for example and, when you are older, become a doctor because that's what they wanted for (or from) you. In this instance it is easy to see the influence of others over your choices. But suppose that you hate your parents or are afraid of them so instead of becoming a doctor you become a 'free spirit' instead, a 'hippie' who travels the world to show your parents that you are not like them and will not be controlled by their wants and desires. Instead, you will impress them with your own adventurous spirit and your ability to live your own way. The point is, though, that you are *still* being controlled by them and far from free because in this case your entire life and not just your career is a choice you made *because* of them. So in this sense can we ever be free?

'Of course as individuals when we undertake an action from some motive we imagine that in exactly the same circumstances we could have chosen to do something else. We do not think we act of necessity. But, as Hume notes, if we try to prove our absolute liberty by doing something 'unpredictable' then we are still acting from a straightforward motive: our motive is the desire not to be seen to be acting from predictable motives,' as Craig Ross remarks. Which, of course, makes us entirely predictable once our pasts and our patterns are known. I imagine, for example, that my client who saw herself as a 'free spirit' is even now repetitively seeking new highs and sexual liaisons, in her mind running towards new adventures and freedom, while at the same time doing exactly what she's always done, not breaking out of her comfortable box of habits at all or, heaven forbid, confronting the things that actually scare her and ensure she keeps running.

What are the implications for society? Well, suppose you commit a crime – in your desire to be free, for example, of the parents who have tried to control you, you steal money to buy that first plane ticket out of here and away from your family home. Who should really be standing in the dock when you are caught? You? Or the father who hit you and caused this chain of events? Who should society punish? Given that our actions are, when looked at in this way, out of our control in any case, should there even be a punishment?

True freedom means being existentially responsible for our

lives. Real freedom therefore comes from commitment – another of life's paradoxes. But can we ever be truly, existentially, responsible or commit to anything while so much of us remains not-us and unknown? Once again, how do we wish to live, and what are we prepared to do to *really* be free? Or will we be content to lie to ourselves and pretend that this faux freedom, this illusion of adventure which is really escape – the ability to get on a plane and keep running instead of confronting our fathers – is *real* freedom; that our pasts, our fears, and all that has shaped us does not matter? That was Sahara's dilemma but maybe it is the same for us all.

Zen Masters have looked at these questions too, as deeply as Western philosophers, and their solution is almost childlike in its elegance and simplicity (since, in the words of the Tao itself, 'the greatest wisdom seems childish'): when it comes to life, *it is what it is*.

To be content with what we have we must let go of the struggle to understand. We can keep asking questions if we wish, just for the joy of asking, but we should not expect answers because there are none. Accepting life for what it is – even if we are in prison and don't even know our jailer – is the only real solution, because wishing it was something else will only cause pain to ourselves and others.

Compatibilism – the idea that we are free and not-free at the same time – is literally true – we are both – but it doesn't help us. What matters is our choices. Do we choose to *live free* (no matter where that choice may actually come from or the fact that freedom itself is illusory) or do we choose to accept that we are conditioned and determined, an option which may in fact bring us more comfort since then we do not have to be responsible for our choices at all?

To be conscious as a human being means that these questions must be considered – but they may as well then be forgotten, since our desire to ask questions at all came from somewhere and where it came from is probably not-us. It is another of Salvia's wheels-within-wheels. The point of life, it seems, is to live it and hope that, at best, we learn something from the experience when it's done.

The Reality Machine

A number of people remark that, as well as entering a 'metallic' and 'alien' space with Salvia, they are at some point in their journeys confronted by a 'reality-making' machine. Deidre's, in Peru, was a reality *annihilation* machine, one that caused worlds to end as the landscapes it contained rolled off the end of its conveyor belts and were swallowed up by oblivion. My client John in Spain, by contrast, encountered a *purification* machine which seemed to give people a new start, so they were reborn from it and 'there were no patterns' in their lives. The artist Bruce Rimmell, in one of his works, depicts a reality *creation* machine, similar in look actually to Deirdre's except it is there to give birth to life rather than end it.

Perhaps this machine really exists? Perhaps, that is, if we are all computer code, what Salvia is showing us in a symbolic way is the computer or games console which houses us and the bits and bytes of information it holds coming into existence, ending, being assimilated and transformed. In this way, perhaps Salvia is simply making the reality of our 'lives' apparent to us?

Even if this is so, however, on another level it also gives us a precise metaphor for who we are as individuals and our particular patterns: the unconscious forces that drive us. This in itself is healing as an insight into our 'sickness' because once we know our disease we can find the medicine that will cure us. In fact, it is even more than this since we are also given a prognosis for where we will end up unless we change our reality. Salvia is, after all, a diviner's plant, able to show us the future.

Bruce, for example, is a creative artist with a number of new projects coming to fruition, including a book and exhibitions of his work. His 'machine' represents a creative force which gives birth to new existences. John, meanwhile, had joined me for a healing retreat when he had his vision, and wanted to free himself of addictive patterns and social anxiety. He sees a purification machine, a hopeful symbol which signifies a new beginning for him free of old 'patterns'. Deidre on the other hand has a long history of endings in her life, including leaving home at age 17 (her earliest opportunity), a series of temporary and part-time jobs that she frequently left, and a string of love affairs that went nowhere, partly because she was afraid of making herself open and vulnerable enough to commit to them. Her longest relationship had been for just three years and she was 'relieved', she said, when it ended. Her reality machine was about death, destruction and endings, a clue maybe to where she is at and, sadly, where she is going.

'Salvia simply shows you where you are,' Dale Pendell writes. 'If you're in darkness, you fly through darkness.'

As a means of escaping that darkness, however, what we are shown can be very useful indeed. As the philosopher Gurdjieff wrote: 'To escape from prison you first need to know you are in a prison.'

'That's what happens when you seize control of the machinery that generates reality. Reality becomes whatever you want it to be,' as Dennis McKenna points out.

Hexagons

Hexagons were prevalent for me and my companions during my first journeys with Salvia in Peru[16] and many other people notice them too, as if the air is filled with them. At first I thought they were just Salvia's peculiar way of painting reality, but I gained further insight into the meaning of the hexagon as a symbol during my third Salvia diet.

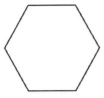

As a form, the hexagon also says something about the human condition, our life journey, and the choices we make. If we imagine ourselves in the present moment to be standing at the mid-point on the left, for example, we can see that we are faced with a Y-shaped moment of choice or possibility, where the universe 'bifurcates', to use the physicist Michael Talbot's word. Our future (and, through our interactions with others, *the* future) is therefore currently unwritten but we will create it in a mere moment by the next choice we make.

Saying yes or no to any possibility at this point (even in answer to the most mundane of questions) will take us in one of two directions (either 'up' or 'down') – and there is no possibility of not choosing since even a decision to abstain is also a choice we are making. Going up or down then confronts us with another Y-shaped point or moment of choice, and so on. And this is what life is: a series of choices we make from the possibilities we create or which are offered to us.

Note, however, that the hexagon is a closed form. By traversing it, therefore, all of our choices (whether we have initially gone 'up' or 'down') bring us back to where we started. No matter what we choose, nothing really changes because of where we began our journeys in the first place. 'Wherever you go, there you are', in the words of the old adage.

In a way, then, the hexagon illustrates the gravitational forces at work on human beings (whether 'cosmic' or, more mundanely, social and familial): the inertia-drag, that is, of our conditioning, habits, 'principles' and beliefs. We may be offered the most amazing opportunities, for example – for personal growth, self-awareness, healing or adventure – but there is something in us (some fear, pride, or the grasping for life of 'old habits dying hard') which still wants to drag us back to our most base conditioned selves.

Salvia offers us the possibility of liberation from this cycle of saAsāra; this boring repetition of self. It shows us our story – the beliefs we have about ourselves and the indoctrinations which form our sense of identity; the parasite that feeds on us and leads us to make the same choices no matter what new possibilities are offered: my client Anton's desire to be 'fulfilled' for example (see next chapter), along with his fear of entering the 'interdimensional doorways' to a new universe where that might actually be possible, or Deirdre's 'annihilation machine' which can only be used to create endings (compared, for example, to John's 'purification machine' or Rimmell's 'reality creation' machine); her desire to 'escape' from where she is, that is, but only as far as where she has always been.

More positively, however, people do not typically see a single hexagon in their Salvia visions, but a roomful.

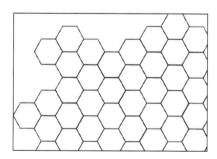

This is a more hopeful symbol since it illustrates the true structure of the universe as 'a void that is also full' (to quote another of my participants – again, see the next chapter). We have an infinity of choices, that is – a virtual web of decisions we can weave for ourselves – and the possibility for change is therefore ever-present. If we are prepared to confront the inertia-drag and, knowing ourselves a little better through work with plants like

Salvia, make more informed and less fearful choices, we can create new patterns for ourselves from literally billions of Y-shaped moments.

This is the intelligence, and the paradox, of Salvia at work again through the symbol of the hexagon: the shape wants to complete itself, to be a discrete and ordered form, just as the universe itself seeks balance and we seek order from chaos in our lives. But we can also do something about that if order leads to predictability and predictability to self-limitation. We may not have the power as individuals to challenge the entire natural order but if we are prepared to courageously face our demons *we* can change, which amounts to the same thing.

We are free and not-free all at once. That may be the meaning of the hexagon.

Zen Paradoxes

Of all the plants I have worked with (and as the above may have suggested), Salvia is the one that most evokes a Zen sensation – the experience of paradox in the union of opposites. Despite her seeming cold, for example, the spirit of Salvia is also kind, telling you cleanly and directly exactly what you need to know. A form of tough love, I suppose. Despite her apparent distance, she is also the only entheogen I know that fully *possesses* you, mind and body, in order to guide and to teach.

While other teacher plants advise and inform, Salvia gives you the absolute truth in a language so clinical it could be mathematics. But even this, in a curious way, engenders a warmth of feeling and a sense of gratitude because it is like having the world's best consultant or cosmologist at your side who has chosen to take an interest in *you*.

The paradox is there in other ways too. The Salvia journey may take you to the void, for example – the vast field of nothingness at the heart of human existence – revealing the ultimate meaninglessness and pointlessness of life. And yet, it is from this field that all things may be created by us. In Bobby's words: 'The Void... was also completely full, a paradox that seemed to be the very essence of Zen.'

Our own paradoxes are often revealed by Salvia too, showing us those unconscious forces which motivate us towards self-harm and which, when finally seen, seem so utterly stupid.

At a workshop in 2012, for example, one of my participants was a woman who had been repeatedly sexually abused by members of her family. Later, to escape from home, she had taken one of the few routes open to her and become a prostitute. She had put that behind her now and was training with me as a healer. One issue she wanted to free herself from, however, was a repetitive pattern of attracting the 'wrong type of man'; one who regarded her as a sex object instead of a human being. Having dealt with her past, what was it about her, she wondered, that still invited such men?

As soon as she smoked she began to panic and I went over to help. Some residual part of her consciousness must have at least recognised me as a man – in fact, as Everyman – because she began screaming at me to leave her alone. At the same time, however, she was grabbing my arm and almost pulling me on top of her. That paradox or contradiction between the words she spoke and the actions she used was the crux of her issue and in just seconds, with in-your-face honesty, Salvia had answered the question that had puzzled her for years and led to her relationship problems. Saying 'no' but meaning 'yes' (or perhaps genuinely meaning no but not having the faith or belief in her own power to really make a refusal) was the issue she needed to deal with; an insight worth years of therapy but delivered in seconds by Salvia.

Love and Karma

J D Arthur describes Salvia as 'almost without feeling', a point I have also made. This absence of love – not quite lovelessness but disengagement from the illusions and projections which usually accompany it – is itself a paradox, for, when we return from our journeys to the void where we have experienced no-love and no-thing-ness, we realise just how precious true love is, unencumbered by the nonsense that often goes with it, as well as the pure acceptance and appreciation of our lovers for who they are and what they give us instead of what we want from them. To be in the place of no-love is to know the importance of real love.

This has ties to another Salvia motif: the realisation that karma is not just a new age theory but a very real force in our lives; that we are connected to everyone and everything and need, therefore, to act in an appropriate way towards all we encounter *because it is us*. Put simply, if we relate to life in a way which is not in the spirit of love, we will attract those same unloving energies to ourselves.

A Philosopher's Plant

Salvia, as you see, is, in the words of Dale Pendell, 'a philosopher's plant'. It raises questions about the nature of life and reality which few of us ever think to ask and even fewer have found a definitive answer to. As Epictetus concluded, in the end it comes down to attitude. In the middle of this great mystery which we call 'life' and accept as if it was real and mattered, how do *we* want to live? What brings us happiness? Because, in a universe of nothingness filled with the potential for anything, everything is available to us. We just have to want it badly enough, believe that it is possible and know that we deserve it. If we choose principles over love, for example, or sickness over health, that is what we create and through it we give to ourselves what we will always get. Our belief in it makes it real.

'The world is as you dream it', as the shamans of the Amazon say; a point echoed by many others, including Shakespeare's Hamlet: 'There is nothing either good or bad, but thinking makes it so', and the scientist, John Lilly: 'Whatever one believes to be true *is* true or becomes true in one's own mind, within limits to be determined experimentally and experientially. These limits themselves are, in turn, beliefs to be transcended.'

3

Healing with Salvia
'Some Sort of Brain Surgery was Performed on Me'

When you study natural science and the miracles of creation ...
if you don't turn into a mystic you are not a natural scientist
Dr Albert Hofmann

Working with teacher plants is like joining an academy of advanced learning and, like the professors in any academy, each plant has particular skills, talents and areas of expertise. Salvia shows us the nature of existence, for example, while ayahuasca teaches us about the creative possibilities of the universe and San Pedro educates us in how to be human.

But that is not all that plants do. They belong to the plant *kingdom* as well, just as every professor, no matter what his speciality, is also a human being and shares characteristics in common with everyone else through his humanity. Plants are the same, so everyone knows something about all others and can teach us about them as well as itself.

Finally, all plants are aware (as some humans, and even some professors may be) that they are ultimately part of the 'mind of God' – or, in quantum language, one expression of the same energy that makes up the entire universe – so they can also open doorways for us into a wider understanding of life. There are four levels, then, of healing possibility with every plant:

1: The Plant as a Medicine

Used in the same way that any herbalist might, Salvia can treat stomach problems, rheumatism and depression, among other conditions. Pharmaceutical drugs derived from the plant could also, as we have seen, be used to combat diseases including Alzheimer's, AIDS, leukaemia and diabetes.

Used in this way Salvia addresses the 'nuts and bolts' of the body; the material stuff that modern medicine and medical herbalism also concerns itself with. Modern medical treatments, however, are based on rather primitive ideas of direct causality and cure – i.e. that A leads to B, or that giving a patient Medicine X will clear up the disease in 96.4 percent of cases – while shamanism also gives attention to the attitude, motivation and psychology of the patient, and to the spirit of the plant.

The notion of magical illness and cure is an example of this and raises, again, questions about the nature of reality and disease. For example, *panzón de Borrego*, as we saw earlier, is a blockage in the stomach (seen as a stone put there by a rival) which may arise because of *mal d'ojo* – giving someone the 'evil eye' because you are jealous of them in some way.

The person who receives such an attack is, of course, a victim of sorcery – but that does not mean that they are entirely innocent since they might in fact have provoked their misfortune by bragging about their wealth or success to others and making them feel bad. Even though they are on the receiving end of negative energy, therefore, they may also be part of its cause. Orthodox medicine or herbalism might well be able to cure the *symptom* of the disease but by ignoring the 'magical' component of the illness it would leave the *cause* untreated and so invite a recurrence. Nor would it offer suggestions for the patient's continuing good health by recommending, for example, that he acts in a more dignified manner in future so as not to provoke the ill-will of others. Used shamanically, however, Salvia can be used to divine the cause of the problem and find an ongoing solution to it as well as an immediate cure. Even from a purely herbal perspective, then, the medicinal use of Salvia is more far-reaching and holistic than orthodox treatments and includes aspects of psychology, counselling and pastoral spirituality.

The idea of magical illnesses and cures (even from this more psychological perspective) is often met with cynicism by Western doctors and sceptics, but it may only be the terminology which offends them because 'magic' itself is used extensively in modern medicine. They just have a more scientific (and, therefore, more seemingly valid) name for it: the placebo effect.

In modern usage, the placebo (Latin for *I will please*) is a simulated medically ineffectual treatment which is given to patients to deliberately deceive them into wellness. Common placebos include inert tablets, sham surgery or false procedures based on what the medical profession calls 'controlled deception'. In a typical case, a patient is given a sugar pill and told that it will improve her condition. Because she *believes* this there is often a real improvement despite (or, rather, because of) the lie she is told. The researchers Wampold, Minami, et al, in their paper, *The Placebo is Powerful* (Journal of Clinical Psychology, 2005) conclude that placebos – the power of belief alone – can, in fact, exceed the effectiveness of 'real' treatments by 20 percent in some cases.

There are also some conditions where pharmaceutical drugs can't be used. For example, burn patients who are experiencing breathing problems cannot usually be given morphine to alleviate their pain as this can cause respiratory failure. In such cases placebo injections (of saline, etc.) are often used, and provide *real* relief when the patient believes that she is being given a powerful painkiller.

The use of placebos by general practitioners is widespread in fact. A study of Danish doctors found that 48 percent had prescribed a placebo at least ten times in the past year. An American survey of more than 10,000 physicians showed that 24 percent would or did prescribe placebos, while a 2004 study of physicians in Israel found that 60 percent used placebos. *The point is that they work. We are capable of curing ourselves.* The last study was reported in the British Medical Journal, the accompanying editorial concluding that, 'We cannot afford to dispense with any treatment that works, even if we are not certain how it does.' (Which is, in a sense, the essence of magic: it works but we don't know how.)

Brain imaging shows that placebos have real organic effects too, causing changes to the brain in the anterior cingulate, prefrontal, orbitofrontal and insular cortices, amygdala, brainstem and spinal cord, among other areas – which is another way of saying that belief – a *non-material* 'substance' – has an effect on our *material* selves. In terms that a shaman might use, *the condition of the body depends on the condition of the soul.*

In fact, therefore, the processes of medical science are sometimes not so different from the healing approach of shamans and demonstrate again that reality is no simple matter. It does not exist 'out there'; it is *created* by *us*. Whatever we believe to be real *becomes* real by the power of belief alone.

2: The Plant as a Spirit Ally

Beyond their purely medicinal uses, plants can teach us about ourselves, reality, existence, and the wider patterns of our lives. To some extent this comes down to what shamans call intention or focus or 'having a good concentration': entering into a committed partnership with the plant with the express intent that it will reveal certain information to us or pass on certain powers, and that, for our part, we will pay close attention to the signs that it sends us and the changes it makes to our bodies in order to receive its messages and gain mastery of the new abilities it gives us. The shamanic diet (see below) is likely to be part of this arrangement.

When intention and attention are used in this way – when we accept that 'nature is alive and is talking to us. This is *not* a metaphor', in the words of Terence McKenna – then anything can become a source of information or power. There are cases of shamans predicting the future by fire-gazing, for example, or reading the shapes in clouds and shadows or observing the flight of birds, but plants are considered to have a special ability to open doorways to other worlds and to enlighten us so that we can, individually and collectively, evolve. As we saw earlier, McKenna believed that some plants (mushrooms, Salvia etc) may in fact have been sent to Earth deliberately by an advanced alien race as a form of communication device. The purpose of this is protective and developmental: to speed our evolution so we can move beyond the 'ape consciousness' of our petty human concerns (war, poverty, ecocide, religious, sexual and social prejudice, etc) and take our place in the cosmos alongside other species who have, perhaps for millennia, enjoyed the freedom of the universe which our own small-mindedness and lack of imagination have prevented us from.

The shamanic diet is the usual process for making an ally of a plant. Anthropologists Schultes and Winkelman defined the diet as, 'A tool helping to maintain the altered state of consciousness which permits the plant teacher to instruct, provide knowledge and enable the initiate to acquire power.' It is a way of releasing the ego and quietening the mind so that the dieter can take on the personality of Salvia and communicate with it in dreams and quiet reflections and then in everyday life.

At first your sense of the Salvia spirit within you will be small and may seem metaphorical or symbolic rather than real, but as the plant establishes itself and the connection between you grows, it will start to be felt more physically, as well as spiritually, mentally and emotionally until it merges fully with your consciousness and becomes 'just there' (as my client John put it during his Salvia diet), like an aura or a shield around you. It is at this point that the plant begins to communicate proactively, offering advice when it is needed and not just when asked for in ceremony.

The diet which achieves this involves certain actions and inactions, including restrictions on the behaviour of the dieter so he can learn from his ally and prepare for the expansion in consciousness that Salvia brings. Foods such as pork, fats, salt, sugar, spices, condiments and alcohol are prohibited, leaving the apprentice with a bland menu so he is not overwhelmed with flavour and can more finely sense the plant. It also weakens his attachments to routines, some of which revolve around meal times and foods. For the same reason there is a prohibition on sexual activity since sex is another worldly distraction and during orgasm we can also give away the power that has been building within us during the diet, which would be a pointless waste.

Breaking these taboos can lead the plant to turn against you so that it takes from you not only the power it has given you but any similar power you may already have had. In the case of Salvia, for example, since the plant's intention is to teach us about the nature of true reality, breaking the diet before it is complete can lead to the opposite of expanded awareness and a clear perspective on life – that is, to madness, according to a warning that Diaz received from a Mazatec shaman.

Diaz was told that his first Salvia diet should last sixteen days, with subsequent diets for a minimum of four days. Since there is little standardisation in the Mazatec approach, however, (for example, in terms of ceremonial etiquette or the number of leaves to be taken in ceremony – see chapter one) I have always followed the Amazonian approach instead with all of my plant diets, including Salvia, and found that it works perfectly well. This lasts for fourteen days. The Salvia is made into a tea with 30 pairs of leaves added to hot water and the infusion left to stand overnight before it is drunk first thing in the morning. The leaves are then chewed and swallowed. The tea is drunk in this way for three days while food restrictions (see above) continue for seven days in total.

At the end of this week a little lemon, salt, sugar and onion is eaten to formally break the diet and provide a safe boundary to the experience while offering protection to the plant so it can continue to grow inside you. There is then an after-diet for a further week and although the same restrictions apply to sex, alcohol, pork and strong spices, other foods can be eaten.

The Plant Diet

Days 1-7: No pork, fats, salt, sugar, spices, condiments, fruit (especially lemon and lime) or alcohol. No sex. Remove yourself from distractions (friends, family, music, TV, books and other media) as much as possible and sleep or meditate as much as you can on what Salvia is teaching you.

Days 1-3: Salvia is taken as a tea made from 30 pairs of leaves added to hot water and left to stand overnight. Drink this first thing in the morning, leaving two hours before anything else is eaten or drunk. The leaves can also be chewed and swallowed.

Day 7 (evening): Eat a little raw onion with lemon, salt and sugar to formally break the diet   .

Days 8-14: Food can be more liberal but still avoid pork, alcohol and sex. Continue to watch your dreams and meditate to hear what Salvia is telling you.

Day 14 (evening): The after-diet ends and eating can (if you wish) return to normal, although some people regard the diet as a form of detox and choose to continue with a new healthier lifestyle.

The biggest challenge for a Westerner undertaking this diet is often not the prohibitions themselves but accepting that plant consciousness can be experienced at all. We are born into the social paradigm that surrounds us with its beliefs and myths and the institutions which support its view of the world, and it is not within ours to easily accept that other beings (plants, spirits, animals) have souls or intelligence and are capable of teaching us anything we don't already know. As we embark on the diet then, we often need to question some of our most deeply ingrained assumptions and to allow that other forms of reality are possible.

For shamans this is not such a problem since, for them, the world we perceive through our senses is just one *description* of a vast and mysterious unseen and not an absolute fact. In his book *People of the Sacred Waterfalls,* for example, Michael Harner writes that for the Jivaro tribe of the Ecuadorian rain forests, '*the normal waking life* is explicitly viewed as 'false' or 'a lie' and it is firmly believed that truth about causality is to be found by entering the supernatural world, or what the Jivaro view as the 'real world', for they feel that the events, which take place within it, underlie and are the basis for many of the surface manifestations and mysteries of daily life.'

Mazatec shaman Maria Sabina said much the same: 'There is a world beyond ours, a world that is far away, nearby and invisible, and there is where God lives, where the dead live, the spirits and the saints. A world where everything has already happened and everything is known. That world talks. It has a language of its own.'

The language of this world is what we learn through the diet.

3: As a Guide to the Spirits of Other Plants

Once it is a part of him the plant ally begins to teach the shaman about itself, about other plants and about how to heal (Mazatecs believe, for example, that Salvia will carry the apprentice to the 'tree of knowledge' in Heaven, where all healing plants grow and where saints and angels will instruct him in their uses). Since all plants are part of the same kingdom, that is, they have an affinity with all others and know something about the specific powers of each. Salvia as an ally, then, is more than just a healer in its own right, it becomes for the shaman a guide to the spirit world in general and an ambassador which will act on his behalf and introduce him to other plants. In my book *Drinking the Four Winds*, for example, I talk about a long shamanic diet I did with the San Pedro cactus and how, during an ayahuasca ceremony to meet its spirit, it introduced me to a number of others that it wanted me to diet, including tobacco, rose, the Amazonian plants jergon sacha and chanca piedra, and Salvia, which is how I came to begin my Salvia apprenticeship (a story told in another of my books, *Shamanic Quest for the Spirit of Salvia*). In this way the shaman becomes knowledgeable about a range of plants and their healing uses and has a guide in Salvia that he can call upon to lead him to those he needs to heal any patient, even if he is unfamiliar himself with the patient's illness or the plants he may need to help him.

4: The Plant as Gateway to the Void, Where We Learn the Deepest Secrets of All

We explored this aspect of Salvia in the last chapter where we looked at some of the themes that emerge through journeying with it. Perhaps the greatest of these is that there is nothing to the universe except what we make it. In this sense, *we are God*, but there is something else – some other force or entity which is beyond us and which, perhaps, will always remain unknown.

In this section I present examples of some of the healings conducted by Salvia which, in most cases, incorporate all of the elements above.

John (a private healing retreat client who dieted Salvia with me in Spain)

When he first smoked Salvia as part of a diet to help with problems related to social anxiety, John felt an immediate impact. 'Some sort of brain surgery was performed on me', was how later he described it, where he became aware of 'the karmic circle of thoughts and how they get trapped in my head. There was something chaotic in my head that needed to be worked on. It was painful, being awake on the operating table, but that passed too. I realized that billions of thoughts are floating around us all the time, and we can cherry-pick them. When we choose one to latch onto we take ownership of it and then *it becomes us*. With Salvia objectiveness it is easier, if that thought doesn't serve us, to just pick another.'

He became aware, that is, of how thoughts *actually* create reality – for example, that he would become anxious before entering a social situation and, as a result of that, think and act clumsily when he got there, so creating a 'real' anxiety. To deal with this he would drink to soothe his nerves, but this usually led to more problems as he got drunk, and therefore to further anxiety. Eventually, something which did not originally exist (since there was nothing to be anxious about before he left the house for his social engagement, as it hadn't yet even happened) became something real purely though the power of his imagination. This is what he meant by his 'karmic circle of thoughts': he was trapped in a loop of unhelpful thinking and action.

What he realised through Salvia, however, is that there are billions of thoughts floating around us and we can choose whichever we want. (*We* create our universe moment by moment through our choices). Once he understood this it was easy for John to dismiss his anxiety altogether by breaking his usual circle of thoughts. In fact, on the last night of his diet a film crew arrived from England to interview me and record our ceremony, and John led some of it. For a young man with a history of anxiety just a few days before to be leading a ceremony on camera was a big step forward.

Anton (a participant on my *Plant Spirit Wisdom* workshop)

Anton joined me to heal a long-standing problem with depression and feelings of inferiority, sometimes leading to suicidal thoughts. He looked terrified as soon as he smoked

Salvia and it seemed clear that the plant was taking a very direct, even confrontational approach to his healing. In response, Anton became confrontational too. He stood up; using his hands to scrape some invisible substance from his arms and legs. (He explained later that he was trying to remove a 'new order of reality' that he saw engulfing his body). He then began speaking to me in a demanding way (there was certainly nothing 'inferior' about him now). I stood up too and held eye contact but did not interfere with his process.

'Reality was immediately cut in half,' he said later. 'I was [cut in half] too and a new atomic universe took hold of my right side. I was afraid and began to try to tear it off me. Ross was not Ross, it was just a name he called himself. I couldn't even say he was human. I began speaking, asking, Who opened the interdimensional gateways? Then I became the guardian of those gateways and was trying to stop Ross, saying, No, you can't enter. This is playing with fire. It scared me to realise how small this reality is and how thin – like a crust around something that contains all we know.'

It seemed to me, in fact, that Salvia was showing Anton his beliefs about himself: the limitations he had allowed to engulf him in his life, 'like a crust' beneath which there was something bigger and much more powerful. He agreed. 'There was something more [and] it was fathomless. The nothingness I saw was full...

'I felt better when I went outside to look at the stars and I was in awe of the sky. The beauty I saw was indescribable. Flowers blossomed from my heart and I felt Salvia as an ally inside me. She gave me a new sacred name. Today I feel I love everyone. My intention was to be fulfilled and I am.'

The outcome of his journey was that Anton felt a greater connection to everyone, and on their level too, not as inferior to them. He was able to see the beauty of the world, and of himself as part of it, and to feel love and fulfilment. These feelings were in many ways new to Anton and perhaps only the first steps on his path to recovery (or, more accurately, *rediscovery*), but they were also real and immediate and they gave him something powerful and positive to build from.

Alex (a participant on my *Plant Spirit Wisdom* workshop)

The second she smoked, Alex staggered across the room to another mat but she couldn't lie still when she reached it. She was extremely agitated, screaming and begging us to 'get me out of here'.

'It was a living nightmare,' she said next day. 'I *became* wallpaper in my family home but not on a wall, on the floor, and I was stuck with my family. My Salvia experience was like a conspiracy they had organized against me. My parents are dead now but I have one sister I don't speak to: they always disliked me and thought I was mad because of my spiritual beliefs, and it felt like this experience was something they'd arranged so I would finally see that they were right and I was mad. I tried to pull the wallpaper off me but it was stuck, and as I pulled at it, it began to tear my whole body apart. I saw that Debs [my assistant] had become the same wallpaper and began to claw at her, trying to get it off her too, and she was also ripping apart. I was shouting, 'Get me out of here.' I felt betrayed by my family: they thought I was mad and wanted me to see what madness was like.'

Before she smoked, Alex's question to Salvia was a simple and practical one: should she leave Greece where she was currently living and move to the UK. She hated Greece and felt she was suffering from being there but didn't feel comfortable in leaving her family and friends. After her Salvia experience she realised, however, just how much she was limiting herself and how illusory her thinking was: 'Part of me wants to stay because of the sense of security it offers but I know now that it is a false security and I have no family there who would ever take care of me anyway'. In reality, her parents were dead and her sister wouldn't speak to her, but in her fantasy she had a loving family; she had been prepared to stay where she was and to damage herself in the process simply to live an illusion.

This case, as good as any, illustrates the difference between orthodox medicine and shamanic healing. A Western doctor might simply have prescribed Alex anti-depressants to deal with her current issues, or some other drug to quell her anxiety (and, indeed, they had done so in the past) but this would not have addressed the real problem or revealed its cause. Salvia did so in minutes and still gave Alex the choice as to what *she* wished to do about it, but now from an aware and responsible viewpoint. As Pendell said, is there any more direct than Salvia in showing us the truth?

As an addendum however, even though Alex's entire mantra during her Salvia journey had been 'Get me out of here' – a pretty obvious answer to her question you might think – she is still in Greece. Once again: we are given information and choices – even direct and obvious answers – but what *we* choose to do with them is up to us.

Commonsense would suggest that human beings use whatever freewill they have to act in their own best interests, but the fact is that they quite often don't. They behave self-destructively instead, or in ways which harm others – it seems just to be a drive we have towards drama and death – and then justify or excuse their actions by reference to 'principles' or life stories and patterns. This is also what Salvia teaches: the madness of human beings and of what we take to be 'real life'. Which in turn raises questions (as we have seen) about just how free we really are.

Michael (a participant on my *Plant Spirit Wisdom* workshop)

Perhaps something similar was going on for Michael. His intention with Salvia was to 'know his spiritual purpose'. On his journey he saw himself as 'an insect trapped on a huge cog, which was rotating, going round and round'. It finally came to rest at a place where there was a plank in front of him and he could step off the cog if he wanted 'but it seemed easier to stay where I was'. Like Alex, Michael was given the information he needed to stop going round in circles, along with encouragement to change his life and his destiny but he decided to stay where he was instead, against his own best interests and expressed intent.

'Then I was in a temple and a group of religious men – sheikhs I think – were talking about someone who had left their order. 'We miss him,' they were saying, 'He was part of us.' Then I was on an airplane and my attention was drawn to another sheikh, but I was told that I shouldn't look at him or be in that part of the plane because an alien experiment was taking place. I didn't believe it but then I was directed to look at a deep incision that the aliens had made in his side. As soon as I saw it the sheikh flew into me. My last recollection was the sound of a gong, like a wake-up noise, then a friend appeared and started telling me who and where I was.'

The fact that a sheikh holy man, 'flew into' Michael is a healing in itself – a change of energy on some level which gave him the potential to find the purpose he was looking for. Once again, however, this is immediately mitigated by the arrival of a 'friend', an old familiar who began telling him who he was; pulling him back to his old identity. The programming in us sometimes runs deep.

Marla (a participant on my *Plant Spirit Wisdom* workshop)
Marla's intention was to become more balanced and achieve her potential. The Salvia seemed to have less impact on her and she felt that she was able to 'observe my own reaction to the whole process'. Later, she commented that:

I was very concerned that I hadn't smoked it right because

I had no great visions or psychedelic effects but then I realized that I was speaking, except my words weren't words. And I had the sensation that I was in two places at once, and that I wanted to be [in both places simultaneously], so *something* was happening. My body was filled with pins and needles and reality became metallic, matrix-like, as if it had been programmed on a computer.

I understood that I wanted to be in two places at once because I had lost so much of my life to depression and I wanted to make up for it. I wanted to share my experience immediately with others as well and I realize now that was because my parents had never listened to me. They always wanted me to do things in the 'right' way, and [because of this] I wanted to check with others to be sure I'd had the 'correct' Salvia experience. I have never been certain that I'm OK and good enough. I have always needed confirmation and security.

Again it seems obvious now (but during the Salvia journey it is very easy to miss the 'obvious', which is why a period of quiet reflection is important afterwards) that Marla's desire for balance had to do with her childhood experience of her parents, symbolised in her journey by her need to be in two places at once; that is, to please her mother and father at the same time who, it transpired, often had opposing views and rarely took her into account. '[They] never listened to me.' During her Salvia journey her overriding concern had been to know that she'd had the 'correct' experience (even though there is no 'correct' experience) – i.e. whether she had done the 'right' thing or been 'good enough'.

Unlike her fellow participants Marla received no wild visions – hardly any visions at all, in fact, except of a reality that was cold and metallic (no doubt symbolic of her family home) – 'as if it had been programmed on a computer' – but nor did she need them because the experience of her journey *was* the message. From it she learned more about the roots of her depression and gained insight into why she wanted to be 'in two places at once'. To understand this and then let it go was the first step for her in achieving the potential it was her intention to find.

Lela (a participant on my *Plant Spirit Wisdom* workshop)

Within seconds of smoking Lela began to moan, then she started crawling across the floor and making slow sideways and forward rolls, head over heels. Eventually she stood and walked unsteadily to the door. I followed her outside where, still standing, she began spinning, arms out at her sides, repeating the words, 'Mother [Salvia], what did I do wrong? Ross, what mistake did I make? Please forgive me, forgive me.' I stayed with her throughout her journey to make sure she was OK.

She said later, during our guidance session, that, 'I didn't notice the transition from this world to SalviaWorld, but then I was flying over the room seeing it like I was an aerial camera... I saw circles, which joined together and became 8s, with the top and bottom rotating in different directions. I felt myself being circles. Who am I? I remembered I had a relationship and a life but then the circles came back and consumed all that. I realized that circling is no fun. In the centre of the 8 I was whole again, and things were still. Then I could see that inside the circles were lots of different life scenes, and I could join any of them.

'I asked Salvia how long this would last. The plant said: *It is infinite*. I asked what the point of it all was. Salvia said: *None*. I was standing up by then and asked if I had done something wrong. Salvia said: *No*. But I started to say sorry anyway... I also remember asking 'Why is this so painful?' and 'Why a baby?' but I don't remember the answers.'

At this point I interjected to ask a question that I thought was central to the story that Salvia was telling her, 'Why did you need to be forgiven?' She began to cry.

Some years ago I was pregnant and I lost the child. I was asking Salvia why ['Why a baby?'] and what I did wrong. Salvia said: *Nothing*. I asked what the point was of this loss and Salvia said *There is no point*. When I asked for forgiveness the plant answered *There are no guilty people and there is no reason for anything*. I have a strong mind and am driven to find the reason for everything; there must always be a solution, but Salvia said *There are no answers to find*. I felt better from this. I knew it wasn't my fault that my child had died.

What I got from the circles is that we can experience the whole of life from the void before we are even born so there really is no point to life or birth because we can stop the circles at any moment where we already are and perceive the realities they contain. We don't even need a body…

In the morning I went into the garden, and I could talk to every plant. I knew its destiny. The day before I had watered these plants but I knew now that it really wouldn't make any difference. The plants had… chosen their own lives so I couldn't change the thoughts or the fate of them or anything else. But still *I* can make a choice to do whatever I want, to water them if I wish… All of life is ultimately pointless and unnecessary but it is an adventure we can have and enjoy.

Lela lost her child many years before this journey and had no conscious awareness now of continuing emotional pain because of it. When she joined the workshop, however, she had physical problems which she wanted to heal and was also very unemotional and 'in her head' (As she said: 'I have a strong mind and am driven to find the reason for everything'). What her example shows, therefore, is how deeply we can repress our pain and shame (our need to be 'forgiven') and the impact on our total body system when we do so – the physical pains which can result, as well as the suppression of emotion and a sort of disappearance into our minds so we are not fully present or whole. It also shows how deep Salvia will go to find a solution, how direct the plant is in finding it, and how quickly it heals. By the next day Lela looked and acted as if a weight had been lifted from her. She had learned – at an emotional level, rather than through her mind (which was her usual way of responding to the world) – that there was no point to her loss, no answers to seek, and that there was no need for guilt or forgiveness either: *There are no guilty people and there is no reason for anything.* She knew then that 'it wasn't my fault that my child had died'.

With this more relaxed, philosophical perspective, she began immediately to come back into alignment, enjoying the garden, for example, instead of feeling a need to water every plant; accepting that 'I couldn't change the thoughts or the fate of… anything', but that 'I can make a choice to do whatever I want' and that while life is indeed 'ultimately pointless' it is still 'an adventure we can have and enjoy'.

This new worldview was a massive shift in Lela's consciousness and, once again, is worth years of more orthodox psychotherapy (an approach which may even have been counter-productive to Lela since it often takes us further into our thoughts and memories instead of our feelings) to get her to this state of *emotional* connection and simple enjoyment of life.

In Lela's example, then, as in some of the others above, we can also see the different levels at which plants heal: as a medicine which has a straightforward and positive effect on the body; as an ally, showing Lela a new part of herself (a repressed emotion, personality or drive that she had kept hidden from herself); as a guide to other plants, leading her, as a form of therapy itself, into a deeper connection with the garden and to a more philosophical instead of a 'mechanical' relationship with the plants there; and finally, as a doorway to new understanding, revealing the deepest truths: *that there is no point to life – and that's OK.*

The Salvia Message

Healing with Salvia, then, often comes back to the same message: that there is no absolute reality, that our life stories are exactly that – *stories* – and that the first essential for positive change is to make new choices based on greater awareness and a decision to embrace love rather than fear.

4

Conclusions and Cautions: Working Responsibly with Salvia

Make no mistake about it – enlightenment is a destructive process. It has nothing to do with becoming better or being happier. Enlightenment is the crumbling away of untruth. It's seeing through the façade of pretence. It's the complete eradication of everything we imagined to be true
Adyashanti[17]

If by 'enlightenment' we mean having our eyes opened to the facts, the cold, hard, truths of the universe and of ourselves, there is no better ally than Salvia. As I have said a number of times, however, it can be an intense and frightening experience because it is so radical and real. There is nothing 'fluffy' about it and it does not concern itself (on the surface at least, and in its immediate effects) with 'love and light' or any other new age concept and platitude; it is reality laid bare in all its horror and beauty.

Even if we are familiar with other entheogens (or perhaps, *especially* if we are), we will most likely be unprepared for the impact of Salvia because the questions it raises are deeper, more significant and more immediate than the other entheogens show us. Perhaps our age demands such swift and to-the-point directness since we seem intent on creating problems for ourselves arising from the 'ape consciousness' of those who lead us, and we are running out of options for their solution. We need answers fast and, Salvia gives us these answers – starkly, directly and unavoidably – to shock us out of our trance.

On top of this directness, Salvia has a language of its own which can be hard to understand. Maybe we need to evolve a little more to read it. J D Arthur called it a 'language of dreams'; I see it as a fusion of mathematics and poetry. It does, however, make the alien landscapes you often find yourself in during a Salvia journey doubly strange and more difficult to navigate because the signposts are not in a familiar tongue.

None of this, however, is any reason not to work with Salvia – quite the opposite, in fact. Just because you don't know the Spanish culture or language doesn't mean you should never visit Spain. By going there at all you have a better chance of learning about the country than by staying safely at home where you never have to try. All pioneers and explorers have, after all and by definition, gone to unfamiliar lands. If they hadn't, we would still be living on a flat Earth and have never set foot on the Moon. Pushing back boundaries and finding new frontiers is how our race evolves – which, in one way, it could be argued, makes it our *duty* to explore and expand our consciousness so that evolution takes place at all. If we are not prepared to do that, then we are just tourists here; freeloaders who are willing to let others do the work for us so we are pulled along in their wake without much effort on our parts. We cannot complain about the world we get if we never put our own energy into shaping it.

There is a difference, however, between conscious exploration and blind, dumb risk-taking, between taking sensible precautions and rushing headfirst into a potentially dangerous unknown. In this chapter I want to suggest some precautions.

What are the Risks?

At the time of writing, there has only been a single death worldwide which is remotely connected to Salvia (compared, for example, to 40,000 deaths in the UK *each year* from alcohol alone and 114,000 from cigarette smoking – see http://www.bbc .co.uk/sn/tvradio/programmes/horizon/broadband/tx/drugs/sur vey/). Predictably, however, it is this single death which has created a moral outcry from the media to have Salvia banned and, predictably again, led to a number of politicians jumping on this bandwagon who haven't a clue about Salvia but do know what gets them votes.

The *facts* are these. In January 2006, Brett Chidester, a seventeen-year-old student from Delaware took his own life by carbon monoxide poisoning. There was no Salvia at the scene and he had not smoked at the time of his suicide. His parents argued, however, that the death of their son was caused by Salvia-induced depression, having discovered the journals he kept of his journeys, one of which included his observation that 'existence in general is pointless'.

Although Brett's statement wasn't made directly in reference to Salvia it is fair to say that it is the kind of truth that the plant does lead us to (it is also one that philosophers for millennia have agreed with). Its ability to state the existentially obvious, however, is no reason to blame it or ban it. (In fact, my view is simple: *There is no justification in banning any substance, even if it is a pure poison* – a charge much more easily levelled at commercial cigarettes or alcohol, by the way – *provided it is taken as a matter of informed personal choice.*)

Nevertheless, bandwagon politics being what they are, as a result of Chidester's death, *Brett's Law* (Senate Bill 259) was passed in Delaware, making Salvia a Schedule 1 substance in that state, alongside heroin and LSD; an event which prompted attorney Alex Coolman to comment that, 'It's remarkable that Chidester's parents – and *only* Chidester's parents – continue to be cited over and over again by the mainstream media in their coverage of the supposed 'controversy' over the risks of Salvia divinorum.' It is worth noting that in the same year as Chidester's death, in Delaware alone, there were 148 fatalities from drunk-driving, 79 gun deaths, and so many deaths from prescription drugs in the USA as a whole that the Center for Disease Control referred to it in their report as an 'epidemic', yet there has been no serious suggestion in Delaware or anywhere else to ban cars, alcohol, guns or prescription drugs.

Update: Just prior to this book going to print I also became aware of one other death has more recently been linked to Salvia, that of Ryan Santanna, a 21-year-old film student from Roosevelt Island, New York.

Santanna smoked Salvia in the presence of a girl friend, Benazir Balani, on the balcony of his fifteenth-floor apartment. Balani said that Santanna then lay down on his stomach and pretended to swim like an animal. 'He stared at me but it was like he wasn't seeing me; it was just a blank stare,' she said. Then he jumped. 'He just ran and hopped over the fence. He had no idea who he was, what he was doing.'

While there is a correlation here – smoke/jump – we do not know what the intervening factors were (if any), such as Santanna's mental or emotional state at the time. The police say he had no history of mental problems. His death, however, is being investigated as a possible suicide. The city medical examiner, meanwhile, said the initial autopsy was inconclusive. Santanna's father is calling for Salvia to be banned. (Source: New York Daily News, March 8, 2011.)

At the very least Santanna's death suggests three of the key precautions I would recommend for any Salvia journey:

1. Know what you are getting into. Salvia is not 'just a legal high' or a 'recreational drug'. *It is the most potent naturally-occurring hallucinogen on our planet* and needs to be treated with respect.

2. Ensure that the setting (the environment around you) is safe and conducive to a Salvia journey and never, under any circumstances, I would suggest, smoke Salvia on a fifteenth-floor balcony where you could easily trip and fall.

3. Always have a sitter with you who knows Salvia, is aware of what you've taken and can help you practically and

emotionally through any difficulties you might have. (Also see my other recommendations later in this chapter.)

So – apart from the natural grief of the parents involved here and our tendency to want to blame someone or something (often, anyone or anything) for our suffering – why the attention to Salvia? Two deaths is, admittedly, two too many, but compared to fatalities from prescriptions drugs, medical care, or the use of recreational drugs like alcohol and tobacco, for example, it is still a very small number.

The 'Experts' Speak

One answer, sadly, is that the 'discovery' of any new 'drug' makes a good horror story which media 'experts' can use to bolster their profile and boost their ratings and salaries. This is the real horror story, in fact: not that 'drugs' exist or that they may need to be used with caution, but that disinformation can be presented to us so easily as knowledgeable opinion and facts. We can, in a way, excuse the ignorance of the general press and our elected repre-sentatives (since we usually, rightly, expect little else from them) but to claim an 'expert' status and then deliver sloppy shock-laden stories is disingenuous in the extreme. Three examples of this are the popular American daytime TV hosts, Dr Drew (http://www.youtube.com/watch?v=nchvRH5ZrL4), Dr Phil (http://www.youtube.com/watch?v=wX8-Pzq85U4) and 'The Doctors' (http://www.youtube.com/watch?v=I0hcKReN5jg). All of them use fear and drama to offer 'warnings' rather than useful information about Salvia and all of them have their facts wrong.

In the first of these clips Dr Drew tells us that he has seen someone drink a small cup of Salvia tea (he indicates the amount with his hands) and 'go into a three-day encephalopathy... it's bad'. The literal meaning of encephalopathy is 'a disorder or disease of the brain', such as Creutzfeldt-Jakob – or 'mad cow' – disease (also known as Bovine Spongiform Encephalopathy). If this were true it would be the first ever recorded incident of anyone getting an instant brain disease from Salvia (or any other herbal tea), despite thousands of trips and almost 100 years of known Mazatec use.

Even if Dr Drew is confusing his words here and he really means that he has witnessed someone undergoing a three-day hallucinatory state from drinking Salvia, this is so unlikely that we can immediately dismiss it as exaggeration unless he has had a *very* unique experience.[18] A tea of the leaves, in my direct experience and that of people who have dieted Salvia with me, is a gentle trip with less potency than smoking a joint of cannabis. It is not drunk to 'get high' (if that is your sole intention, drinking the leaves will prove a waste of your time) but for spiritual self-reflection, and your journey with it will last around 30 minutes, not three days. I doubt that this 'expert' has any real experience with Salvia at all, and certainly none of his own.

In the next clip, Dr Phil tells us that Salvia is, 'like LSD but anyone can just walk in [to a head shop] and buy it,' a line which he delivers in a way that makes LSD itself sound like the work of the Devil. While it is true that salvinorin – the concentrated extract, *not* Salvia itself – is gram-for-gram *stronger* than LSD, the trip lasts for minutes rather than hours (even with concentrates of 100X, the longest salvinorin journey I have had or witnessed was around 25 minutes, and most people will smoke extracts at far lower concentrations than that). Furthermore, the trip itself is nothing like LSD (Ketamine, if we needed one, would be a better analogy). It seems apparent therefore that LSD is mentioned solely for its shock value and is not meant to serve any useful purpose in educating people about what Salvia actually is or does.

Finally, there is The Doctors clip, where a volunteer purports to smoke Salvia on camera so we can see how it affects him. He then tells us, quite lucidly, how his 'trip' is progressing, inter-cut with concerned looks on the faces of audience members, while another 'expert' dressed in a blue surgical uniform for no useful reason except to appear like a 'medical authority' gives us an 'objective' and 'scientific' commentary on how the volunteer looks and feels: 'wobbly' apparently (as if this would not be obvious and expected and a cause for little concern from anyone who has taken a mind-altering substance, including a few shots of whisky). The 'Salvia trip' shown looks and sounds like no other I have seen or experienced at *any* concentrate level. In fact, by virtue of the fact that the volunteer can describe his experiences at all (or even think and talk coherently), it suggests that he has taken so little Salvia that he is in no position to make any serious comment about its effects.

On the other hand, those who actually *have* tried Salvia and have a more informed story to tell (and therefore more claim to the title 'expert') have usually done themselves no favours either. A search for the word Salvia at YouTube for example produces over 200,000 results, but they are mainly of kids making idiots of themselves, putting themselves in danger, and giving media 'experts' and politicians another reason to call for the plant to be banned – which is self-defeating and stupid, even if your intention is only to have fun with a 'legal high'.

From this evidence, the biggest risk with Salvia is not death or three days of 'encephalopathy' but having an 'expert' use your party clip to make a name for himself. Minimising even this risk is simple enough, however. It just needs attention to set and setting.

Set

The term set refers to the state of mind with which you approach your encounter with any teacher plant.

Personally, I do not believe it is possible to have a 'bad trip' with any entheogen, in the sense that there is anything contained within the plant itself which is deliberately out to show us disturbing images. All entheogens are there to teach and as part of that process they may show us things that we have repressed and would prefer not to see, but these things are already within us; they are not visions which the plant has imposed on us from elsewhere. The point of showing them to us is so that they can be known, brought to consciousness and dealt with, and their energy released since, hidden or not, these things are already within our psyches and driving us in ways that we cannot control.[19] It is only when we become aware of them that we hope to exercise any freewill over our destiny.

The most important practice for avoiding the completely unexpected and finding yourself face-to-face with a part of your unconscious that you are not yet ready to see is to set an intention for your journey.

Intention provides a road map and a framework for the trip you are about to take. It gives it direction and purpose. Going into a journey without intention (especially with Salvia) means that you are likely to be plunged quickly into chaos, with fast-moving images which make no sense to you and leave you overwhelmed, panicked and confused. Having a *reason* for taking the journey, however, (for example, to explore the outcomes of a decision you are about to take – i.e. divination) means that everything you see, hear or feel relates to something definite. It may still feel chaotic at the time but in the context of your intention even the chaos may be meaningful.

To set this intention it is useful to have a quiet time of meditation or reflection before you journey in order to clear your mind and focus on what you want to achieve. Shamanic plant work is never recreational, it is purposeful; it not about getting high but getting answers. Focus leads us.

Once your journey begins it is unlikely that you will remember your intention – or much else (you may very likely not even remember who 'you' are). J D Arthur writes about this too. 'It was suggested in some recent writings that one should hold a question or similar thought in mind while entering the [Salvia] state...

'As I began to enter the state [however] it became obvious that... in an ironic twist [I] would have to relinquish my ordinary thought processes, which, of course, was precisely where my question resided. Without the footing of thought there could be no question. It just didn't seem possible to bring the camel with me through the eye of the needle.'

The solution to this is not to fight your loss of self or to try to hold on to your intention during the initial parts of the Salvia journey but to let it go. In shamanic terms, intention alerts the spirits to our purpose so they are aware of the reason for our visit (like setting the agenda for a meeting) but we do not have to continually refer to it once they have been informed.

It is after we return from the journey that we begin the work of decoding the symbols presented to us and this is when we refer to intention again. Taking 30 minutes of quiet reflection time after the journey ends means we can return gently to the 'normal world' and look again at our purpose. We can then interpret the information we have been given within the framework it provides so that our images make more sense.

To aid the focus on intention the diet (see above) is useful since this is the means of making an ally of a plant and forming a definite bond with it. It is also a commitment to the journey. If you don't want to follow a full diet, however, at the very least (to avoid the possibility of sickness if for no other reason) it is best to forego all food for about eight hours before your journey and take no liquids from about two hours before. Since Salvia journeys are usually at night, this means eating nothing after lunch and if your ceremony begins at, say, 9pm, drinking nothing from about 7pm. It goes without saying that the taboo items on the shamanic diet – alcohol, pork, lemons, salt, spices, sex, etc – should be avoided altogether. These things are excluded for good physiological as well as spiritual reasons as part of a procedure which has been practiced by shamans for thousands of years.

Ignoring their advice is not something you want to do with a plant like Salvia.

Setting

Setting refers to the environment and circumstances in which Salvia is taken. In all shamanic work, ceremony and ritual precautions are essential since you will be dealing with spirits and energies which are otherwise uncontained. The results of this can be unpredictable at best, dangerous at worst.

Always ensure that Salvia is taken in a safe, calm, quiet space, in darkness, away from other people, noise and distractions and with a clear intention in mind. This is basic commonsense and spiritual etiquette. Taking Salvia to show off in front of friends is asking for trouble on all sorts of levels, including psychologically, emotionally and physically. It *is* highly advisable, however, that you have a sitter with you – someone sober, sane and sensible who knows Salvia but does not smoke it at the same time as you so they can take care of you, prevent you from hurting yourself (for example, if Salvia compels you to move) and give you emotional support if you find yourself in a challenging situation. Ideally, your sitter should also be able to talk to you with good sense and insight after your journey ends as this is normally helpful in providing you with greater clarity on your experiences. They should therefore be someone you trust to offer you sage reflections and keep your secrets as you will literally be bearing your soul to them.

If you are smoking Salvia in a pipe, do not cram it with leaves. Start small, even with one or two, and build to higher doses as you gain familiarity with the plant and its effects and get to know your tolerances.

If you are smoking salvinorin you can also do so in a pipe on a substrate of leaves or tobacco. *A few grains are literally all you need.* Do not imagine for a moment that 'this tiny pinch of salvinorin couldn't possibly have an effect on me' and be tempted to add more. This is the world's strongest natural entheogen and we are literally measuring in micro units. People who have experience with other hallucinogens but have never smoked Salvia find it hard to believe that so little is needed, but trust me on this.[20]

Keep your lighter flame in the bowl of the pipe as you inhale.[21] Two or three inhalations are probably the most you will manage and all you need. Again, don't be tempted to overdo it.

Your sitter should then take the pipe and the lighter from you and encourage you to lie down and remain as still as possible throughout your journey. You may be unable to stop yourself moving, however, and your sitter should be aware of this. They should follow your movements, intervening only when necessary (with words or actions) to prevent you from hurting yourself and, other than that, remain a quiet, unobtrusive, supportive presence throughout.

The foregoing should be considered the *basic* precautions for working with Salvia in any situation. If you wish to work shamanically with the plant, however, you will also want to introduce a more formal ritual aspect. This is to form a bond with helpful spirits, to alert Salvia to your intention to work with it, and it also gives you a useful psychological boundary to assist your work and enhance your safety by providing the session with a definite beginning and end.

My own procedure is to set up a *mesa* (an altar containing *huacas*: 'power objects', ritual artefacts and items of spiritual significance from sacred sites I have visited, each of which has importance for me). I then make a silent or spoken prayer to the spirit of Salvia and the other helpful spirits I wish to watch over the ceremony, and to the seven directions of east, south, west, north, above (Heaven, the sky), below (the Earth) and the centre where, symbolically, I will sit, so I am protected on all sides. I then 'seal' the entire space with a rattle to keep it pure. Following that, I extinguish the candle and begin.

If I am running the ceremony for others I do not take Salvia at the same time as them, although I usually smoke it first in their presence to show them what to expect. This means that I am able to assist them, one at a time, to smoke, and everyone else in the room is instructed to remain silent and pay attention. When everyone has smoked and been allowed 30 minutes or so of reflective silence, we all come together in circle to discuss our experiences. I offer feedback and everyone is allowed to contribute in a calm and helpful way, reflecting back what they saw and heard to the person whose journey we are discussing.

At the very end I offer a prayer of thanks to the spirits who have watched over us and release them from our ceremony. Diaz' shaman, don Alejando, would also at this stage bathe participants in a cold water infusion of Salvia leaves in order to break their trance and bring them fully back to 'normal reality'. I rarely do this as I prefer my participants to stay slightly in Salvia space so they can go to bed when the ceremony ends and take more guidance from the spirit of Salvia in their dreams.

Rituals gain more power when they are personalised, so that you invest yourself more deeply in them, but this is a framework you could adopt for your own explorations.

The Legalities of Salvia

The legal situation regarding Salvia is subject to change so it is wise to keep an eye on things yourself. At the time of writing, however, Salvia is legal in most countries, although there are varying levels of control in America, Australia, Belgium, Canada, Denmark, Estonia, Finland, Italy, Japan, Russia, Spain and Sweden.

Australia and Italy have made Salvia a Schedule 9/Table I controlled substance, for example, (both US Schedule I equivalents), while in Spain there are controls only on the sale of Salvia and personal cultivation is allowed, and in the United Kingdom there are no controls at all.[22]

In America, legislation for amendment of the Controlled Substances Act to place salvinorin and Salvia in Schedule I at the federal level was proposed in 2002 but failed. Some American states (now including Alabama, Delaware, Louisiana, Michigan, Missouri, Ohio and others) have passed their own laws, however, and others (including Alaska, California, Florida, Iowa, Maryland, New Jersey, New York, Oregon, Pennsylvania and Texas) have proposed legislation, although many proposals have not made it into law, and where they have the degree of legislation varies from state to state.

The concerns of politicians and law-makers tend to directly reflect those of the media (the blind leading the blind), with comparisons to LSD and outraged appeals to 'protect our children' being parroted from media to political pulpit. Legislative proposals tend to follow news stories therefore – which is another reason not to give the media more ammunition by posting videos of Salvia experiences – so it is worth keeping an eye on the papers for mentions of the plant.

On a more informed and rational level, those who are *genuinely* knowledgeable about Salvia advocate consideration of its *full* potential (i.e. its beneficial uses in a modern context as well as the cautions that may be needed when using it) and argue that more could be learned from Mazatec culture, where Salvia is not associated with drug-taking at all but is considered a spiritual sacrament. Some doctors (as we have seen) are also excited by the diseases that Salvia may target. We must hope therefore that good sense prevails over 'expert opinion', but that also depends on us treating Salvia seriously and with respect and maintaining a non-sensationalist profile in regard to our own discoveries.

Final Words

As with all work in shamanism and with plant teachers in particular, it is impossible to simply read about the experiences of others and believe that we understand it or can apply the lessons of these teachers to our own lives. As J D Arthur puts it: 'Without some type of direct experience of the transformative nature of substances such as Salvia shedding light on the genuine fallacy of the validity of our normal perceptions and revealing hints about the true nature of the perceiver, any differentiation of the real from the false will remain in the realm of words alone.'

The way to really *know* Salvia therefore is to go in search of her yourself. But do not expect to return from SalviaWorld the same person who entered it. This is both an encouragement and a warning.

Endnotes

1. 'Don' is a title which means something like 'doctor'.
2. See later in this book.
3. It may well have been a UFO actually, as this seems more usual in the experiences of my participants. See later in this book.
4. See for example the other books in this series on ayahuasca, San Pedro and magic mushrooms.
5. See, for example, http://www.washington.edu/news/2012/ 12/10/do-we-live-in-a-computer-simulation-uw-researchers-say-idea-can-be-tested
6. See http://www.youtube.com/watch?v=q1LCVknKUJ4
7. *Who Built the Moon?* Watkins Publishing, 2011.
8. See my book *Shamanic Quest for the Spirit of Salvia* for other accounts and for background to the reports given here.
9. See my book *Ayahuasca: The Vine of Souls* for a fuller description of Kira's journey.
10. See *Is it Possible to Change Reality?* Wonderpedia, February 2013.
11. David Suits is professor of philosophy at Rochester Institute of Technology, New York. His quote is from *Body Snatchers: The Invasion of Philosophy* in Philosophy Now magazine, January 2002.
12. The X nominally represents a multiplication of strength so that a 5X extract refers to a concentrate that is roughly five times stronger than a normal dose. The reason that this is nominal, however, is that nobody quite seems to know what a 'normal' dose is, as we saw in the last chapter.
13. There is more advice in the final chapter on how to develop intention and the importance of having a reliable sitter with you as you journey.
14. See my book *Shamanic Quest for the Spirit of Salvia* for a fuller

account.

15. See the next chapter for more on this.

16. See my book *Shamanic Quest for the Spirit of Salvia* for further detail on this.

17. Adyashanti (born Steven Gray in 1962) studied Zen for fourteen years and, at age 25, began experiencing a series of spiritual awakenings, the nature of which he described as 'liberation from the sense of an 'I' or of a 'me' trying to be happy'. In his philosophy 'enlightenment' is informed disinterest in the quality or experience of life: a sort of 'who cares' attitude. As such, for example, it is possible to be 'enlightened' (whatever that means beyond an awareness of the simple truths of life) and still experience anger, depression, regret, envy, hatred, sorrow, grief, etc – a view which diverges considerably from the one that many (including those in new age spirituality and traditional Buddhism) have long held about enlightenment: that it is about finding happiness, love and compassion, etc. Adyashanti's view corresponds more closely to the teachings of Salvia: that life is essentially meaningless and existentially pointless. It is what we *make* of it – and however we *choose* to make of it what we will – that gives it meaning. Since Salvia is, as I've said, a 'philosopher's plant' that very often evokes similar Zen-like realisations, Adyashanti's message is no doubt one that the sage would approve of.

18. To my knowledge only one plant in the world might conceivably produce a three-day 'hallucination' from a single infusion of its leaves and it is not Salvia, nor is it easily mistaken for Salvia. And you would have to drink considerably more of it anyway than Dr Drew indicates.

19. See, for example, the case I quoted earlier of the woman who was branded a slut by her father and who set off on sexual and other adventures to escape his judgement by becoming a 'free spirit'. What she achieved, ironically, was a level of

promiscuity which might in fact justify her father's judgement and which led her to situations which were dangerous and actions which were self-harming, such as a case of cervical cancer. If an unconscious drive to 'spite her father' was the point of all this she would, paradoxically, have been better off becoming a nun, although that wouldn't have seemed to her much like defiance.

20. Salvinorin can also be smoked in a bong or vaporised and inhaled or used as a tincture. The pipe however is, in my experience, the easiest method and the safest as long as a sitter is present.

21. Salvinorin burns at high temperatures so a butane lighter is best, but not essential.

22. In the UK, a 2005 parliamentary Early Day Motion was raised calling for Salvia to be banned but it only received 11 signatures. A second motion in 2008 attracted a few more (18 signatures) but still failed. The Advisory Council on the Misuse of Drugs (the independent body that advises UK government) was asked to investigate it further, however.

Moon Books invites you to begin or deepen your encounter with Paganism, in all its rich, creative, flourishing forms.